After the Diagnosis

How to Look Out for Yourself or a Loved One

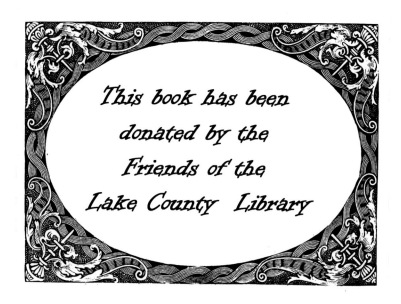

After the Diagnosis

How to Look Out for Yourself or a Loved One

DONNA L. PIKULA, D.D.S., M.S.

Books 2 Help You, LLC
Hartland, Michigan

After the Diagnosis

BY DONNA LEE PIKULA

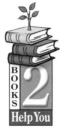

Published by:
Books 2 Help You, LLC
P.O. Box 130
Hartland, MI 48353
www.books2helpyou.com

Definitions reprinted from *Mosby's Medical Dictionary,* 6th ed., St. Louis: Mosby, Inc., 2002, with permission from Elsevier (see References for page numbers).

ISBN-13: 978-0-9768970-0-2
ISBN-10: 0-9768970-0-8

Publisher's Cataloging-In-Publication Data
(Prepared by The Donohue Group, Inc.)

Pikula, Donna L.
    After the diagnosis : how to look out for yourself or a loved one / Donna L. Pikula.
    p. : ; cm.
    Includes bibliographical references.
    ISBN: 0-9768970-0-8

    1. Patient education. 2. Therapeutics—Decision making. 3. Medical care—Decision making. 4. Patient participation. 5. Medical personnel and patient. 6. Patient advocacy. I. Title.

R727.4 .P55 2005   615.5/071

Edited by Gail M. Kearns, To Press and Beyond,
Santa Barbara, California www.topressandbeyond.com

Book and Cover Design by
Peri Poloni, Knockout Design, Placerville, California
www.knockoutbooks.com

Printed in the USA

To my grandmother Edith, *with love.*
Thank you for teaching me that everyone
needs someone looking out for them
at one time or another.

Contents

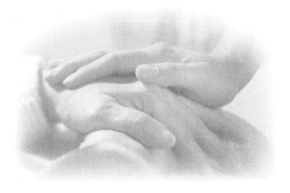

Acknowledgments

I believe there are at least two things in life money cannot buy. One is time. Everyone has a finite amount of it, so when someone shares their time with you it is a special gift. They are *choosing* to share their time with you instead of spending it in countless other ways.

The second thing money cannot buy is life experience. It is something that develops over time and as people age their life experience grows. Everyone has life experiences and no two people ever have exactly the same ones. This is great, because if you choose to pay attention, you can literally learn something from everyone. Someone sharing his or her life experience with you is a very precious gift indeed.

I mention the gifts of time and life experience because in writing and developing *After the Diagnosis*, I've been extremely fortunate to receive both of these gifts from a number of special people.

After the Diagnosis probably would have stayed a beginning manuscript without the guidance of Gail Kearns and Peri Poloni. Gail was the editor and production coordinator for the book. More than that, she was the person who always kept the "big picture" in focus and helped guide me through the long process of turning thoughts into a book others could understand. Thank you for this and your patience. Peri was the book and cover designer who continually came up with ideas I had never thought of, but I ended up really liking. Thank you for your instinctive creativity and your patience as well.

After the Diagnosis is a better book than it started out to be because of the ideas and contributions of a number of people. These people shared their time and life experiences through their comments on the manuscript for no reason other than as a favor to me. So, I would like to wholeheartedly thank: Colleen deBeauclair, Tara Gnau, Nancy Langley, Dr. Stephen Lutz, Marlene Pikula, Linda Siaje and Dr. Peter Stevenson. Thank you for your unselfish contributions.

I would be remiss if I did not thank my family for their understanding, love, and support. To my immediate family, thank you for understanding the countless hours I disappeared to work on this project. I know it was not always easy to have me *missing*. To my parents, thank you for always supporting me in all the different ways you have over the years. I would not be who I am today without having learned from you and your life experiences.

Finally, I would like to thank all of the people not specifically mentioned above whom I have learned from. Without these people I would not have had the idea to write *After the Diagnosis* in the first place or have had anything to say on its pages. You really can learn something from everyone if you take the time to do so.

Thank you again to all involved for sharing your gifts of time and life experience. I will always be grateful.

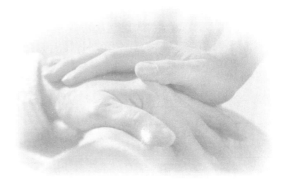

Introduction

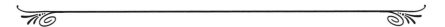

The idea for this book came about because of helping myself and other family members through different health care issues. Some issues were minor and temporary while other issues were severe and life altering. The more severe health issues made lasting impressions on me and influenced the formation of this book.

Like all families, my family has many health stories to tell. One of my family members (a long-time former smoker) was diagnosed with severe emphysema (lung disease characterized by difficulty getting enough oxygen exchange in the lungs) and had to cope with the difficulties of being continuously connected to an oxygen tank for the last few months of her life.

Another older family member developed dementia (mental confusion) and the inability to take care of herself. She eventually ended up in a senior care facility and her personality and physical abilities slowly disappeared as her dementia increased. She spent several years in this facility, which provided an entirely different level of experience for our family. We learned not to be shocked by things like patients wearing each other's clothes and taking things from each other's rooms without each other's knowledge. These events are not uncommon on dementia floors where patients often don't even remember what room, let alone items, is theirs any longer. Even though she was in one of the better care facilities available, we encountered many challenges trying to have her cared for as we wanted her to be cared for. Near the end of her life, she didn't talk much and you were never quite sure if she recognized you or if she thought you were someone else.

Still another family member developed lung cancer and had to learn quickly how to *figure out what to do next*. She quit smoking, underwent surgery and was lucky to get a second chance at life because she was diagnosed before the cancer had metastasized (spread to other areas). She also had the advantage of having found one of the top cardiothoracic surgeons in the country to treat her.

Thinking back even further, there were other family members who I didn't help but who had just as memorable medical stories. A thirty-something family member went into a coma following *routine* gall bladder surgery. It was later discovered that she had stopped breathing in the recovery room while no one was watching her. Several years later, she died in a health care facility without ever waking up. Another older family member walked into a hospital with pneumonia and within a few days was pronounced brain dead because he had stopped breathing and no one found him in time either.

By now you might be thinking that when it comes to health matters, I'm part of a very unusual, unlucky family, but I've had some interesting medical experiences as well. I once was given a totally different drug by a pharmacy than what my doctor had intended.

My doctor had phoned in a prescription for an antibiotic and I was given a muscle relaxant instead. The muscle relaxant would have never fought the infection I had. Luckily, I always check my prescriptions before taking any medication so I was able to discover the drug error and get the situation corrected. However, the interesting thing is that the doctor and the pharmacist both thought it was the other person's mistake. This experience is a great example of drugs, with very different purposes and actions, being confused over the telephone because they have similar sounding names and each person thought they said/heard something different.

I have also had the unfortunate experience of being incompletely diagnosed. I spent months being treated for acid reflux-like symptoms when in reality I had a larger problem — a thyroid gland with an overactive area. This situation went on for several months and I found myself seeing doctor after doctor. They all treated me for acid reflux — a commonly diagnosed problem of stomach acid flowing backward from the stomach into the esophagus — and brushed off my questions asking if my problem couldn't be related to a thyroid condition. There is a history of thyroid problems in my family and my instincts kept telling me my problems were related to my thyroid gland. The doctors continued to tell me I just had acid reflux and I should keep taking "the little purple pill." I couldn't understand how I could *so suddenly* develop acid reflux. After all, I had always been able to eat anything I wanted and now even eating cereal and drinking water made me hurt.

After seeing several different local specialists and undergoing many, many tests, I referred myself to an endocrinologist (someone who specializes in thyroid diseases) at a large medical center for another opinion. Within five minutes of meeting this endocrinologist, he was convinced all of my symptoms were related to being hyperthyroid (too much thyroid hormone). He explained to me that when you are hyperthyroid all the systems in your body are hyper (overworking) and can give you symptoms I was experiencing like acid reflux! I was never so relieved — I had finally found someone who believed that my symptoms were related to a thyroid problem. Further testing confirmed his diagnosis, and surgery was scheduled to remove my thyroid gland. It seems my instincts were right after all. Since having surgery (I now need daily thyroid hormone replacement) my symptoms have disappeared and I no longer need "the little purple pill" for acid reflux. Sometimes you have to keep asking and pursuing answers until a situation makes sense. My only regret is not finding the right doctor sooner. I could have avoided many unnecessary tests and months of suffering.

So now you must be thinking that just my family and I are unlucky or unusual — or that maybe we should try our luck at the lottery. After all, how can so many things happen to *one family*? Incidentally, some of my family members have tried the lottery; they are still waiting for that *one* lucky ticket. The truth is, while the exact number of these types of stories may vary from family to family, all families have members or friends who go through unusual or difficult medical journeys. I'm sure if you think about it, it isn't hard for you to find similar medical situations among your family and friends.

The overriding lesson I learned from all these experiences is that when confronted with difficult medical situations, most people have no idea where to start or what to do next. Most of the time, patients merely try to follow the verbal instructions they receive from their family doctor. They do not know how to proceed any differently and they are given very little written information or none at all. Some doctor's offices are better than others at handing out brief brochures on certain medical illnesses, but step-by-step *how to* written instructions are rarely given unless for a specific medical test. Patients are then often sent on to see specialists who usually require more testing.

Following all the testing, patients are expected to decide the best treatment option for themselves, oftentimes without fully understanding all the words used to describe their illnesses let alone the complex details of their treatment choices and consequences. Doctors' offices are very good at the mechanics of providing treatment to a patient, but in general they are not as good at educating patients or helping patients cope with broader issues following a diagnosis.

Patients are not generally referred by their doctors to resources or associations related to their particular problem. This extra step could really help patients get through difficult times and decisions. Other resources/associations can provide benefits to patients through written materials, websites, support groups, buddy systems, and much more. They are very good at helping patients connect with other patients who have had survived similar experiences. This connection can be meaningful for a newly diagnosed patient. It gives them an opportunity to speak with someone who really understands what they are going through and offers them hope that they too can make it through the challenges. Most of the time patients have to find these other resources on their own, if at all.

My experiences have taught me that I have a distinct advantage over other patients. I have been on both sides of health care delivery. I have been the doctor giving diagnoses and treatment plans and I have been the patient receiving the care. I know how medical care is supposed to work. I know how to look out for my loved ones and myself. I know how to use valuable resources. I know these things because of my medical/dental education and my experiences. And yet as a patient, it took me months to find my own medical answers to my thyroid problems. This just shows that the delivery of medicine isn't perfect and doctors do not always have all the answers no matter how much we want them to. Sometimes the medical journey is difficult because of the nature of the problem, not finding the right doctor, or not being in the right place for a particular treatment. Sometimes, even under the best circumstances medical errors occur that no one can foresee. The study of medicine has also become very complicated and specialized. For these reasons, today more than ever, patients need to learn to look out for themselves. Patients need to take advantage of every piece of medical knowledge, all resources available to them, and work with their health care providers to find their best medical options and treatment. They also need to learn to listen to their instinct — that little voice inside them that tells them whether something seems right or not.

Having survived my own incomplete diagnosis, I began to wonder what in the world do people do who don't have medical training or background? How do they know where to start, what to do next? How can patients make intelligent decisions regarding their health care when they have never been given the education, skills, or tools to do so? After all, navigating the health care system is not taught in public schools. It is from asking these types of questions that the concept for *After the Diagnosis* developed. I wanted to use my knowledge from having been on both sides of the health care system to help other patients learn how to look out for themselves or a loved one. So, I decided to create a book that would be easy to understand, provide basic medical information/resources for all ages, and provide step-by-step guidance/tips that could be applied to all medical problems no matter how minor or severe. Patients could use the information in this book as a starting point upon which they could build their own individual plans to assist them in playing an active role in decision making along with their health care providers. After all, educated patients are much more prepared to play an active role in their treatment.

After the Diagnosis provides basic information about health care, step-by-step forms, and commonsense tips every person and caregiver can use. This book compiles information from many, many different sources into one handy reference book. Reading this book is an excellent way to gain the initial knowledge necessary to better understand *the big picture* after the diagnosis and what you need to do for yourself or a loved one. Through a better and more comprehensive understanding of a particular situation, you will be better equipped to ask appropriate questions, use available additional resources, and make better informed decisions along with health care providers for you or a loved one. All of these skills will increase your chances of a having a successful medical journey.

Thinking about medical problems and situations is not something anyone wants to do, but it is something everyone will have to do at some point in their lives. Medical problems/situations are a part of life — it is inevitable that they will happen to you or someone you know. Wouldn't you rather be prepared with basic medical knowledge and know how to develop a plan *before* you or a loved one is diagnosed? Of course you would! The best part is, you don't have to struggle from square one. You can benefit from my knowledge and experiences and use *After the Diagnosis* to jumpstart your preparation for your or a loved one's medical journey.

Disclaimer

As stated numerous times in this book, the information contained within these pages is intended to be used for educational purposes and solely as a starting place to obtain a better understanding of what to do after you or a loved one receives a medical diagnosis. The information in this book is not a substitute for professional medical evaluation or advice. Rather, the many examples in this book should be used as reference tools to assist you. While this book presents helpful information about how to actively participate in health care, it is impossible for any book to be able to identify you or your loved one's medical problems or to make specific medical recommendations for you or a loved one. One's medical needs, specific treatment options, specific medical care, and specific treatment fees can only be determined after clinically seeking the recommendation of licensed medical professionals.

This book also provides general information regarding payments and medical insurance, but your specific situation may be different from the information presented. It is also impossible for any book to know the particular specifics of your medical insurance coverage and policies. The terms, examples, and tips are best used as a basis for education. One's specific payment plans and specific insurance coverage can only be determined after consulting with specific medical offices, laboratories, hospitals, and insurance companies.

Having stated these limitations, *After the Diagnosis* remains a valuable reference tool for most individuals.

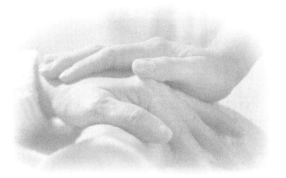

CHAPTER 1

Why You Need Someone Looking Out for You

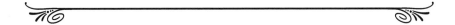

It's Not Yesterday Anymore

In days gone by, there was one doctor in town, and everybody saw this doctor. He took care of them, from the moment of their birth to their children's births and even beyond that. This doctor delivered babies, treated illnesses and injuries, tried to keep everyone healthy, and oversaw care of those who couldn't be helped anymore (until they left this world). The doctor was a neighbor as well as a health care provider, and everyone trusted and believed him and his diagnoses. There was a one-to-one doctor-to-patient relationship that lasted until someone moved away or passed on.

Today, the doctor-patient relationship is different. Instead of one doctor in town, there are many doctors, and the town itself is a lot

1

bigger with many more patients. Both doctors and patients move from town to town more often. While towns have grown, so has the study of medicine.

There has been a great deal learned about the diagnosis and treatment of so many diseases that it's impossible for any one doctor to know all the answers any longer. For this reason, medicine has become specialized. Doctors often become specialists and practice in only one particular area of medicine. This means that the doctor won't be taking care of a person's every need. Specialization allows doctors to keep up with and know the newest discoveries and treatments in their specific areas. Some doctors even hire professional medical readers to review new journal articles and study areas of new research for them. This allows doctors to keep current and still have time to see patients. However, it's impossible for any one doctor to know about all the advancements in all areas of medicine. So, patients with multiple medical needs may see several doctors on a regular basis instead of just one doctor as in the past. Seeing several different doctors can cause confusion for the patient and the doctors themselves if everyone doesn't have the same information or if doctors have different opinions or ideas about treatment.

In addition, patients today are often treated by a variety of health care providers, not just doctors. It's not uncommon for patients to see a physician's assistant or nurse practitioner instead of a doctor. These health care providers have more education/training than a nurse, but less education/training than an M.D. (Doctor of Medicine/physician) or a D.O. (Doctor of Osteopathy/physician). They are often able to write prescriptions and manage certain medical visits on their own. Frequently they will have more time to spend with a patient, but they do not have the same qualifications as a physician. (For more information about medical personnel abbreviations see Chapter 3 — Health Care Provider Abbreviations.) Some insurance plans like to manage clinics with many physician's assistants or nurse practitioners working under the direction of a physician. This management plan saves money for the insurance company that's running the clinic because they have to pay fewer physician salaries. Patients who seek care at these clinics may not realize they're seeing a nonphysician unless they ask. While nonphysician health care providers are valuable assets, patients should always know whom they are seeing and what training/degrees the provider has. Nonphysician health care providers do not have the same education/training as physicians and are not always appropriate substitutes for physicians.

Whether we like it or not, insurance companies have also changed the doctor-patient relationship. As more and more people have medical insurance, insurance companies have played a larger role in how doctors practice. Insurance companies pay doctors for office visits and procedures performed on a patient. Doctors are usually not paid for their time spent on your treatment when you are not there. For example, they are not paid to coordinate your care with multiple physicians or to explain every area of your care in great detail. As a result, doctors tend to see many patients a day for short intervals of time per patient.

A recent article in *U.S. News & World Report* (Hobson, 2005) discusses these issues. In "Doctors Vanish From View," Rachel Naomi, a community medicine professor at UC San Francisco, states, "The average doctor sees 25 people a day. I don't even know how to say hello to 25 people a day." The article also discusses how the "average 17-minute office visit may not be sufficient to get enough information to diagnose the problem and talk about the ever growing list of health issues they're supposed to bring up." This means that the average patient has a meager 17 minutes to discuss all of their needs/concerns with their doctor. Worse yet, "those meager 17 minutes may be with a different doctor every few years, because when employers switch insurers, or people change jobs, their old doc often isn't part of the new plan. That's a real loss. When you aren't familiar with a patient's past care, it becomes difficult to track, monitor, and anticipate the medical needs."

Some insurance companies make it difficult for a patient to see a specialist without first being referred by a primary practitioner (internist, family practitioner, or pediatrician). In fairness, doctors are also human. They only have 24 hours in a day just like the rest of us. However, the reality of today's health care system in the United States is that a patient's primary physician has limited time and financial incentives to see many patients per day. There is no financial incentive for doctors to look out for a patient's total care — even though most doctors genuinely want to do this.

Concerns about the quality of health care in the United States have prompted many organizations to investigate the quality problems and recommend improvements or solutions. One such organization is the Institute of Medicine (IOM). The Institute of Medicine of the National Academies is a private, non-profit organization chartered by Congress to advise the government on health policy advice. Since 1996, the IOM has been assessing and making recommendations to improve the nation's quality of care. As a result of this ongoing assessment, sobering statistics have been collected and reviewed by IOM. The following is a list of these statistics showing significant problems in the delivery of health care in the United States:

❖ Between 44,000-98,000 Americans die (in hospitals) from medical errors annually. (Institute of Medicine, 2000; Thomas et al., 2000; Thomas et al., 1999)

❖ Medical errors kill more people per year than breast cancer (42,297), AIDS (16,516), or motor vehicle accidents (43,458). (Institute of Medicine, 2000; Centers for Disease Control and

Prevention; National Center for Health Statistics; Preliminary Data for 1998, 1999)

❖ Over 7000 people died in 1993 from medication errors: accidental poisoning by drugs, medicaments, and biologicals that resulted from acknowledged errors by patients or medical personnel. (Institute of Medicine, 2000; Philips, et al., 1998)

❖ Medication-related errors for hospitalized patients cost roughly $2 billion annually. (Institute of Medicine, 2000; Bates et al., 1997)

❖ Only 55 percent of patients in a recent random sample of adults received recommended care, with little difference found between care recommended for prevention, to address acute episodes or to treat chronic conditions. (McGlynn et al., 2003)

❖ Forty-one million uninsured Americans exhibit consistently worse clinical outcomes than the insured, and are at increased risk for dying prematurely. (Institute of Medicine, 2002; Institute of Medicine, 2003a)

❖ Eighteen thousand Americans die each year from heart attacks because they did not receive preventive medications, although they were eligible for them. (Chassin, 1997; Institute of Medicine, 2003a)

❖ More than 50 percent of patients with diabetes, hypertension, tobacco addiction, hyperlipidemia, congestive heart failure, asthma, depression and chronic atrial fibrillation are currently managed inadequately. (Institute of Medicine, 2003c; Clark et al., 2000; Joint National Committee on Prevention, 1997; Legorreta et al., 2000; McBride et al., 1998; Ni et al., 1998; Perez-Stable and Fuentes-Afflick, 1998; Samsa et al., 2000; Young et al., 2001)

✤ The lag between the discovery of more effective forms of treatment and their incorporation into routine patient care averages 17 years. (Balas, 2001; Institute of Medicine, 2003b)

These statistics are alarming and much more information about them can be found by visiting IOM's website at www.iom.edu or by locating the references. Detailed information to help you locate references can be found in the Reference section at the end of this book. Taking the time to read the papers and articles will help you better understand how the problem was looked at and what the statistics are based on. As an example of this, the next paragraph discusses more thoroughly the statistic on page 5 regarding the percentage of adults receiving recommended care.

A study looking at the problem of receiving quality health care in the United States was published in the *New England Journal of Medicine* (June 26, 2003). This study looked at the quality of health care delivered to adults in twelve different U.S. cities. The study was conducted through telephone interviews with participants, reviewing the participants' actual medical records, and analyzing the results. Although many different conditions were looked at, the national study found that "overall, participants received 54.9 percent of recommended care." **This means that the participants in this study received the appropriate health care only about half the time.**

While the study went on to say that although "the exact size of the quality problem may continue to be debated, the gap between what we know works and what is actually done is substantial enough to warrant attention. These deficits, which pose serious threats to the health and well-being of the U.S. public, persist despite initiatives by both the federal government and private health care delivery systems to improve care." Although the exact percentage of time recommended health care is received can be debated (due in part to difficulties of conducting such a study), there is no doubt that there are serious problems with the quality of health care delivered in the United States (and undoubtedly elsewhere as well).

The problem of receiving quality health care in the United States is even worse if you are an older American. An article in the *AARP Bulletin* (November, 2003), "Second-Class Care: Discrimination Against Older Patients Still Permeates Nation's Health Care System," discusses the problem of ageism in the U.S. health care system. Ageism is defined in the article as "the term for discrimination against older people coined more than 30 years ago by Robert N. Butler, M.D., the founding director of the National Institute on Aging." The article goes on to discuss the findings from a report by the Alliance for Aging Research, which can be found at www.agingresearch.org/brochures/ageism/index.cfm. In this report ("Ageism: How Health Care Fails the Elderly"), the alliance discusses how ageism in health care hurts older Americans. The report discusses five key areas where health care fails older Americans:

1. Health care professionals do not receive enough training in geriatrics (branch of medicine that treats older patients) to properly care for many older patients.

2. Older patients are less likely than younger people to receive preventative care.

3. Older patients are less likely to be tested or screened for diseases and other health problems.

4. Proven medical interventions for older patients are often ignored, leading to inappropriate or incomplete treatment.

5. Older people are consistently excluded from clinical trials, even though they are the largest users of approved drugs.

Problems in the delivery of health care in the U.S. for everyone, and changes in the doctor-patient relationship, have created a real concern for the average patient seeking care. For example, if a patient is seeing multiple doctors, then who is making sure all of the doc-

> *There are problems for everyone trying to receive health care in the U.S., but older Americans have an extra burden due to the ageism bias against them.*

tors have the same information about a patient, such as medical history, current medications, tests taken, or procedures performed? No one physician is going to be able to coordinate all of this information, so a lot of the responsibility for a patient's own care falls to the patient. The patient (or in some cases a patient's loved one) is expected to keep everything straight and on track during treatment. The patient ends up playing a much larger role than in the past. While it's true that no one will look out for yourself as you would, many patients don't have the education necessary to look out for themselves. Most patients think doctors speak and write in a different language called "doctor speak." How are patients supposed to understand complex medical conditions without understanding *doctor speak*, or without having someone to explain *doctor speak* to them? The answer is that patients and patients' loved ones need to educate themselves so they are better able to make the right medical decisions in combination with their health care providers.

The need for patients to play a larger role in improving the quality of their health care is echoed in an accompanying editorial in the same *New England Journal of Medicine* (June 26, 2003) that reported the study of health care delivered to adults in the U.S. In an editorial by Dr. Earl Steinberg (referring to the study above), he suggests several actions to improve the quality of care for U.S.

patients. One of these actions stresses the importance of patient participation. This action states, "we should draw on the power of patients to improve the quality of care they receive and their health outcomes. We cannot achieve meaningful "consumer-driven health care," however, simply by increasing consumers' financial stake in the cost of that care. To engage consumers and empower them to take increased responsibility for their health and health care, we need to provide them with information about the care they should receive and consider receiving. To be effective, that information needs to be authoritative, easily accessible, easy to understand and to act on, timely, and personalized."

The more health information available to patients and their loved ones, the better off everyone will be. Patients who know more about their health care will be smarter patients, and they'll be able to develop certain skills that will help them to look out for themselves more successfully. These skills can easily be remembered by using the letters S-M-A-R-T. Smart patients:

Today, more than ever, patients need to be better educated about health care issues so they can play a larger role in making important decisions with their health care providers and avoid becoming part of a sobering statistic themselves.

S = Seek help

M = Make decisions, plans, and organize care

A = Ask questions

R = Research and investigate

T = Trust their instincts

You will see many examples of these skills being used throughout this book.

The remainder of this book is meant to provide you and your loved ones with information to help you better understand health care and develop the skills of SMART patients. Please use this information in combination with your health care providers. Best wishes for a successful journey!

The First Step

The first step in looking out for yourself or a loved one is to realize that you have the right and the ability to ask questions of your health care providers. While this may seem obvious to some of you, to others it may be a difficult concept to grasp. How many people do you know who don't ask questions they really want answered because they do not want to question the doctor? Many people who feel uncomfortable asking questions were raised with the idea that the doctor is always right and you're not allowed to question his or her decisions or abilities. If you're one of these people, or if you know one of these people, then the best advice you can be given is — get over the idea that the doctor should not be questioned!

You have every right to ask questions about your medical care!

You should never feel you are bothering the doctor, or that your questions are not important enough to ask. Asking questions is the only way you can start to look out for yourself or a loved one. Answering questions is part of a doctor's responsibility. They should answer your questions or direct you to someone who can better answer your questions if they're not sure themselves. If you visit a doctor that won't take the time to answer your questions, then the problem lies with the doctor — not with you. In this case, you might want to consider finding a new doctor. Having said this, you also need to understand if the doctor asks you to return at another time to more thoroughly answer your questions or if the doctor asks if he or she can call you back by phone. Sometimes you are not scheduled for a long enough appointment time to accommodate all your questions.

Another reason to ask questions of your doctors and other health care providers is that they are human — just like you! Although they try hard to be correct all the time, they make mistakes too. Sometimes errors occur because of a faulty system, process, or condition that leads people to make mistakes or fails to prevent them ("To Err is Human: Building a Safer Health System," Institute of Medicine, 2000). Organizations like the IOM, hospitals, and other health care providers and companies are working hard to try and reduce health care errors. Some examples of these efforts are:

✤ Using bar code technology and sophisticated software to help prevent medication errors in hospitals.

✤ Eliminating certain medical abbreviations in hospitals, which often lead to mistakes in prescription drugs and other medical procedures.

✤ The Food and Drug Administration trying to prevent the naming of sound-a-like drugs that cause the wrong drug to be given.

✤ Surgeons marking the area of surgical incision before patients are put to sleep, so the correct side or area will be treated.

✤ Development and use of standardized electronic health records that would allow multiple health care providers, health care facilities, and pharmacies to share the same individual patient information, thus avoiding information that is incorrect or possibly left out.

While progress is being made and systems are being put in place to reduce medical errors, errors are still occurring at unacceptable rates. Your best chance to avoid becoming an error statistic is to ask questions and be active in your or a loved one's treatment. This is the best thing you can do to help reduce the chances that a mistake will happen or not be caught.

Although it may be hard to do at first, asking questions of your doctors and other health care providers is very important. Take the time to write down any questions you may have before your appointment. This will help you remember all the questions you want to ask and free your mind up to listen more closely during your appointment. Remember, it is your right and in your best interest to ask questions.

The next section will give you suggestions on how to find someone to help you look out for yourself.

Patient Advocate

A patient advocate is simply someone who watches out for your best medical interests. It is someone you trust to help you through medical treatment or tough medical decisions. A patient advocate can help you in many ways. Patient advocates can:

✤ Be an extra pair of ears to listen at appointments. This is always a good idea! Remember, some people are shocked when they receive serious medical news and they may not be able to listen well or know what to do next. A patient advocate at your appointments can confirm what you heard and fill in areas you may have missed.

✤ Take notes at your appointments. This will free you up so you can concentrate more on listening and understanding.

✤ Get you to appointments. Patient advocates may be able to drive you to your appointments if you are unable to drive.

✤ Provide whatever support is needed after surgeries or procedures. This could mean staying with you at the hospital, helping you get your medications, caring for you until you are back on your feet, etc.

✤ Make decisions. A patient advocate can always offer another opinion.

✤ Assist you with needed care or everyday activities.

✤ Simply be there to listen to you.

✤ Research information about your disease or condition.

✤ Find support groups or associations for your disease or condition.

✤ Keep the big picture in mind.

✤ Keep you moving forward. It is important to make forward progress.

Remember, a patient advocate is on your side. They are looking out for your best interest.

A patient advocate can also make decisions regarding your medical treatment if you are not able to do so. And even though no one wants to think about it, it's smart to have someone chosen as your patient advocate before you need them. In order for a patient advocate to act on your behalf, they need legal authority to do so. A medical durable power of attorney is one way you can give someone the legal authority to act on your behalf when you cannot make medical decisions. An example of the need for this would be if you were in a coma and unable to communicate. If you had a medical durable power of attorney in place, there would be no question as to who could make decisions for you. If you did not select someone before you went into a coma, a different family member or even a stranger may have to make decisions for you. These people may not know your wishes. It is important to plan ahead!

You should consult with an attorney to decide the best way for you to give someone the legal authority to act as a patient advocate on your behalf. Your wishes, where you live, and your particular situation may all play a role in deciding what legal paperwork is best for you and your patient advocate. A medical durable power of attorney is just one of several options you and your attorney can choose from.

How to Choose Your Patient Advocate(s)

Deciding on who your patient advocate should be is an important decision. The person(s) you choose may even change over time. When you are young, it may be someone older than you. When you are older, you may choose someone younger — perhaps one of your children. Or, you may alter your wishes because of a geographic location change. Regardless of when or how often you replace your advocate, you need to make sure your decision is also legally changed, when necessary.

The person(s) you choose should be someone you trust. They should also be someone who has the time and desire to help if you need them. If possible, you might want to consider a person who has some medical knowledge. This could be someone who is a physician (not your own physician), nurse, pharmacist, dental hygienist, ultrasound technician, veterinarian, medical office manager, etc. Most everyone knows someone who works in the medical field. Choosing someone in the medical field as your advocate will give you an advantage because they will be able to understand your disease or condition more quickly than someone who doesn't understand medical terms or procedures.

When choosing your patient advocate it's a good idea to choose someone who is not squeamish about watching medical procedures or being in hospitals. It is also good if you can find someone who deals well with the unexpected. After all, a patient advocate cannot possibly know all the situations that may arise beforehand. Having someone who can think on their feet is always an asset.

CASE STUDY

A fairly common example of a patient advocate having to deal with the unexpected involves Kathy, a younger patient advocate, who is trying to help her elderly mother Estelle. Kathy noticed that her mother Estelle had become increasingly disheveled, disorientated, and had more and more difficulty moving around her house. Most days Estelle stayed in her bathrobe, never combed her hair, was unsure what day it was, and had to place her hands on walls or the furniture to steady herself as she walked around. Kathy was concerned about her mother living alone and finally decided that enough was enough. She scheduled an appointment for her mother to see her doctor. Kathy had already told her mother that she was concerned about her living this way and thought they should visit the doctor for help.

> *If you don't know anyone in the medical field to become your advocate, then you might consider someone who is organized and able to learn quickly. Someone who can research your disease for you would be a great help, even if they didn't already have a medical background.*

Kathy arrived early at her mother's house the day of the doctor's appointment, fully expecting that she would have to help her mother get ready. To Kathy's surprise Estelle didn't need any help at all. She was well dressed, carefully groomed, and wearing make-up. Estelle even greeted Kathy with a cheerful, "Good morning"! Kathy blinked her eyes a couple of times to make sure she was really seeing this well-dressed, cheerful woman who looked like her mother — but how could this be? Before Kathy had time to think about what to say next, Estelle had locked her door, brushed past Kathy, and walked on her own to Kathy's car. Kathy, now confused, didn't understand how her mother had gotten so much better when only two days ago she could barely move around her house. It seemed miraculous!

The doctor appointment went smoothly, as Kathy's previously confused and slow-moving mother confidently greeted the receptionist, the nurse, and the doctor. At one point the doctor even asked, "Why are you here?" *Why are we here?*, Kathy wondered. *We are here because my mother has become confused lately and she is having difficultly walking and taking care of herself.* She started to relate this to the doctor, but found her voice trailing off as both she and the doctor looked at the smiling, well-groomed woman seated before them correctly answering questions about time and space. To humor Kathy, the doctor asked Estelle to walk down the hallway. *Now he will see how she really is,* thought Kathy. Both Kathy and the doctor watched Estelle march down the hall and back as if she was auditioning for the Rockettes! Estelle's steps were sure, quick, and steady. Her hands were at her sides, and there was no reaching out for the wall to steady herself like at home. Kathy felt foolish and became quiet for the rest of the visit as Estelle and her doctor exchanged pleasantries. Kathy had just encountered the unexpected. Had a miracle really occurred? Had Estelle really recovered?

The next time Kathy visited Estelle, she was once again greeted by her disheveled, slow-moving mother. Reality had returned and it would take some time for Kathy to discover that when threatened, a patient can do remarkable things. Estelle had felt threatened by Kathy's words and actions. She was sure Kathy was getting ready to put her in an old folk's home! Estelle had a stress reaction to this threat that set off a whole series of events in her body, which helped her *perform* the way she did. This natural reaction is known as the *stress response* or *the fight or flight response*. You may remember learning about it in school. This response allowed Estelle to *perform* well under pressure. For Estelle, it was "showtime"! She needed to *perform* well to be able to keep living alone. After the immediate threat of the doctor's appointment had ended, Estelle's body returned to a more relaxed state and the "miracle" was over.

Kathy and Estelle's story is a common one. Caregivers and patient advocates struggle with difficult issues like these everyday. Kathy, as Estelle's patient advocate, will have to find a way to help her mother and have others see Estelle as she normally is. At times, being a patient advocate can be a tough, thankless job. Make sure you choose someone who is mentally strong and who can go the distance. Similarly, if you are asked to be a patient advocate, realize that at times you might have to be extremely strong and learn how to deal with the unexpected yourself.

While there is no magic formula for finding your patient advocate(s), everyone is capable of finding one. Even if you don't have close family near you, there is probably someone available who would be a great advocate for you. You might consider the following persons as sources for your patient advocate:

- ✦ Yourself (if you are able).

- ✦ Spouse.

- ✦ Child (if an adult).

- ✦ Parent.

- ✦ Sibling.

- ✦ Other relative.

- ✦ Best friend.

- ✦ Church member.

- ✦ Someone with medical knowledge.

- ✦ Organized friend with ability to learn.

- ✦ Friend or relative who doesn't mind being in hospitals.

- ✦ Someone who can think on their feet when dealing with unexpected.

- ✦ A person who is mentally strong and can go the distance when needed.

Close family and friends are the most commonly chosen advocates, but these other options might work for you as well. You may not be able to find someone that meets all of your criteria, but you can certainly find someone who will do an excellent job of looking out for your best medical interests.

Anyone can benefit from having a patient advocate, but it is up to you as to how much you are willing to let this person help you. Some people are very private and don't want to share their personal medical information with anyone unless they have to. Other people rely heavily on others and are willing to share in return for the benefits they receive from involving them.

Your specific disease or condition is also very important when considering how much of a role you want your patient advocate to play. If you have a problem that has been around for a long time and it is merely an inconvenience, then you might or might not involve your patient advocate. However, if you find out you have a serious illness, you probably need to get your patient advocate in your corner from the start.

There is no one right answer for who you choose and how much help you accept from your patient advocate. Everyone and every situation is different. You must make the best choice for you at the time. The important thing is to have a patient advocate chosen and available *before* your diagnosis. The *Patient Advocate* form can be used to write down contact information about your patient advocate(s). An example of a completed *Patient Advocate* form can be found on the next page. The line about the location of legal papers refers to where you are keeping the legal papers that designate who your patient advocate(s) is. You can leave this line blank or fill in as much detail as you are comfortable with. Examples of what you fill in could be: at my attorney's office, safe deposit box, in firebox at home, in safe at home, etc. (For photocopying purposes, a blank *Patient Advocate* form can be found in Appendix 1.)

All of the forms used in this book can be found in Appendix 1. These blank forms are placed together in this section so you can easily photocopy them and fill in the answers appropriate for you. These forms are meant to help you, so please use them!

Patient Advocate(s)

for

IMA Smart Patient

(Your Name)

Effective as of January 2, 2004

(Date)

First Advocate (Primary)

Name: Good Husband

Address: 123 Homesweet Home

Address: Mytown, USA 45678

Phone #: Home # 313-123-4567

Phone #: Cell # 313-987-6543

Second Advocate (Secondary)

Name: Best Friend

Address: 321 Friendship Road

Address: Mytown, USA 45678

Phone #: Home # 313-336-7773

Phone #: Cell # 313-248-6663

Location of legal papers: Safe at home; safe deposit box

Medical Alert Information

Another way of looking out for yourself or a loved one is by having medical information available immediately during an emergency. Think about it: if you are away from home and you become unconscious (due to an accident or illness) how would anyone know important medical information about you? Any health care provider treating an ill or injured person wants to know if s/he is on any medications, has any serious medical problems, or is allergic to anything (especially medications). If the person cannot answer these questions, then the health care provider has a much tougher time trying to figure out what is wrong and what is the best treatment for that person.

Immediate access to medical information can make treatment during an emergency much easier for the provider and much better for you. Drug interactions and drug allergies can be avoided if your information is known right away.

Medical Alert Jewelry

Medical information found with you can be in your wallet, your purse, or on your body by means of a medical alert bracelet or necklace. A bracelet or necklace is a better choice than information in your wallet or purse because it can always be on you. Purses or wallets are

There are two primary ways you can provide important medical information to someone without having to speak. One is through the use of medical information found with you by means of medical alert jewelry. The second is through medical information services provided by a third party. Contact information engraved on medical alert jewelry is used to reach this third party.

often left at home or not with you if you are involved in an activity like swimming. There are companies that can provide you with engraved bracelets and necklaces for a one-time fee per item of jewelry. Your doctor's office or pharmacy often has brochures for such companies. The bracelets and necklaces are usually reasonably priced and have a medical symbol on them in addition to your important information. They can be worn all the time even when swimming or bathing. They should be removed only when absolutely necessary, such as for medical testing or when a job or procedure would make wearing them dangerous. Examples of items that can be engraved on medical alert jewelry include:

❖ Names of medical conditions (diabetes, epilepsy, leukemia, hypertension, asthma, etc.).

❖ Current medications.

❖ Allergies (especially drug allergies or bee sting allergies).

❖ Emergency contact name and/or number.

It is important to decide exactly what information you should have on a medical alert bracelet or necklace. Your doctor should be able to help you decide what medical information is important enough to be placed on your bracelet or necklace. There is a limited amount of information that can be placed on each piece of jewelry, so while you want to be complete, you also need to be as brief as possible. Emergency medical providers are trained to look for such medical alert jewelry. When choosing the emergency contact name and number, try to pick a contact that can always be reached. Don't include someone who doesn't return phone calls quickly. Some people choose their doctor's answering service, while other people choose the cell phone number of someone who always has their cell phone with them.

Companies that provide you with alert jewelry for a one-time fee do not provide any other service except mailing the necklace or bracelet to you. Once you have verified that the information engraved is correct, their service to you is done. Health care providers helping you during an emergency must rely solely on the engraved information if you are unconscious.

Medical Information Services

The second type of immediate medical information available during an emergency uses medical alert jewelry, but in combination

Any emergency medical provider can call MedicAlert's phone number 24 hours a day, 7 days a week, 365 days a year and receive important information about the person wearing their MedicAlert emblem. This is the big difference between wearing an alert necklace and wearing an alert necklace that is connected to a service like MedicAlert. There is always someone available to provide information such as:

* *Specific medical conditions*
* *Medications*
* *Allergies*
* *Implanted devices*
* *Emergency contacts*
* *Insurance information and more*

Regardless of what type of medical alert you use, it is important to remember to update the information. Wearing a necklace or having a link to a medical information service is only as good as the information available to emergency health care providers. Make sure all of your medical and contact information is updated as changes occur. Keeping the information current is one of the best ways to look out for yourself.

with a medical information service. One of the best-known services of this kind is MedicAlert®, a nonprofit U.S. organization that maintains a huge database of information about individuals. MedicAlert was founded by a physician in 1956 and it protects and saves lives by providing identification and medical information in emergencies. MedicAlert also uses medical alert necklaces and bracelets, but engraved on each piece of jewelry is a person's identification number, primary medical condition(s), and the phone number of MedicAlert's 24-Hour Emergency Response Center.

Even though MedicAlert is a nonprofit organization, there are costs associated with setting up the information in each person's medical file and in keeping the information current. To cover operating costs (in 2005), MedicAlert charged a $35.00 enrollment fee for the first year (includes the MedicAlert emblem) with an annual renewal fee of $20.00. MedicAlert can sometimes offer their services to qualifying people who cannot afford the first year's enrollment fee by using donation money. For information about MedicAlert and the services they offer, visit their website at www.medicalert.org or you can call 800-432-5378 toll free.

Deciding which type of medical alert is best for you is a personal decision that depends upon your medical condition(s), and your peace of mind. It is a decision that should be discussed with your doctor. For some people who do not have a serious medical illness, but may have just an allergy, simply wearing a medical alert necklace with the specific allergy on it may be enough. For other people with more than one severe medical problem, having a link to a service like MedicAlert, in addition to a medical alert bracelet, might be the best choice.

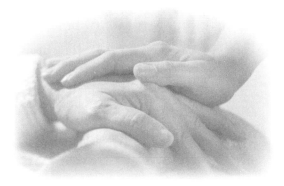

CHAPTER 2

The Diagnosis

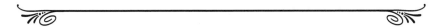

What Is the Disease or Condition?

The next step to looking out for YOU is to know the specific name of the problem and, if possible, a few key words to describe it. This information is important because without it you cannot even start to understand or investigate the problem. This minimal information is needed to decide if the problem is a small difficulty or a serious illness. The definitions for all of the medical terms listed below come from *Mosby's Medical Dictionary*, 2002, unless otherwise noted. A few key terms you should know are:

✤ Disease — a condition of abnormal vital function involving any structure, part, or system of an organism. A specific illness or disorder characterized by a recognizable set of signs and symptoms, attributable to heredity, infection, diet, or environment.

- ❖ Condition — a state of being, specifically in reference to physical and mental health or well-being.

- ❖ Biopsy — the removal of a small piece of living tissue from an organ or other part of the body for microscopic examination to confirm or establish a diagnosis, estimate prognosis, or follow the course of a disease.

- ❖ Tumor — a swelling or enlargement occurring in inflammatory conditions. Also called neoplasm. A new growth of tissue characterized by progressive, uncontrolled proliferation (growth) of cells.

- ❖ Benign — (of a tumor) noncancerous and therefore not an immediate threat, even though treatment eventually may be required for health or cosmetic reasons.

- ❖ Malignant — tending to become worse and to cause death (describing a cancer) — anaplastic, invasive, and metastatic.

- ❖ Metastasis — the process by which tumor cells spread to distant parts of the body. Because malignant tumors have no enclosing capsule, cells may escape, become emboli, and be transported by the lymphatic circulation or the bloodstream to implant in lymph nodes and other organs far from the primary tumor (adjective form is metastasize).

- ❖ Acute — (of a disease or disease symptoms) beginning abruptly with marked intensity or sharpness, and then subsiding after a relatively short period.

- ❖ Chronic — (of a disease or disorder) persisting for a long period, often for the remainder of a person's lifetime.

- ❖ Mild — gentle, subtle, or of low intensity, such as a mild infection.

❖ Moderate — tending toward the mean or average amount of dimension (*Merriam-Webster's Collegiate Dictionary*, 2004).

❖ Severe — of a great degree or serious (*Merriam-Webster's Collegiate Dictionary*, 2004).

❖ Staging — the classification of phases or period of a disease or other pathologic process, as in the TNM clinical method of assigning numerical values to various stages of tumor development (T is for tumor, N is for lymph node, M is for metastases).

❖ Diagnosis — identification of a disease or condition by a scientific evaluation of physical signs, symptoms, history, laboratory test results, and procedures.

❖ Prognosis — a prediction of the probable outcome of a disease based on the condition of the person and usual course of the disease as observed in similar situations.

Many more medical terms and their definitions can be found in the next chapter.

> *Note: For simplicity sake, the reference to "you" made during this chapter and the rest of this book applies to either "you" meaning yourself or "you" meaning a loved one. It is easier to read "you" instead of "you or a loved one" each time. This simplification will apply to all forms of you, your, and yourself.*

The use of medical terms such as these combined with the name of the disease or condition can already tell you a lot about the problem. As an example, there is a big difference between these three diagnoses:

❖ Spot on your face.

❖ Benign keratosis of the skin.

❖ Malignant melanoma of the skin.

The words *spot on your face* do not tell you anything about what the spot is. This diagnosis doesn't tell you whether the spot is something you don't have to worry about or something that could kill you if it is not treated. A diagnosis of benign keratosis of the skin is not bad. The word *benign* helps to tell you this right away. Benign keratosis of the skin is a darker area of skin. Even though you may choose to have the benign keratosis removed, leaving it in place is not a problem that will kill you. On the other hand, malignant melanoma of the skin is a serious problem. The word malignant in a diagnosis is always a concern. For the most part, malignant means cancer. Malignant melanoma is a serious disease that can kill a person if not treated early enough because the disease can spread to other areas of the body (metastasize). From these examples, it's easy to see how knowing just a few extra words can add a lot of meaning to a problem.

Having said this, sometimes when you and your doctor are just starting to investigate a problem, all you may know is that you have a spot on your face. Sometimes more testing is needed to figure out what the exact problem is. For some diseases or conditions, many medical tests are needed. For other problems, like a spot on your face, a biopsy can often give a clear diagnosis. After a biopsy, the spot on your face becomes an exact diagnosis, like *benign keratosis of the skin*. Your doctor can best determine what tests are necessary to help reach a diagnosis.

Other words, like *acute* or *chronic*, tell you how long the problem has been around. Still other words can tell you how far along the disease is; for example, mild, moderate, or severe. Some diseases like cancer are staged to determine how far along they are. There are different staging systems or methods for different cancers, but usually the higher the number, the worse the problem is. For example, lung cancer has four stages with stage four being the worst. It is not unusual for a patient to undergo many different kinds of tests in order to stage a serious disease like cancer. Once a disease is staged, then a prognosis, or prediction, can be made. Though far from exact, this prediction (the likely outcome) can be helpful in making further treatment decisions.

Once you know as much as you can about your diagnosis, it is time to start investigating and asking questions. One of the most important questions you can ask is, "How much time do I have to decide upon treatment?"

How Much Time to Decide?

Once you are diagnosed with a disease or condition you must ask the physician:

❖ How serious is the problem?

❖ How far along or at what stage is the problem?

❖ How much time do I have to decide upon treatment options?

Remember, you may not get the answers to all these questions at one time. Sometimes it can take several visits to your physician before all these questions can be answered. Once you have the answers to these questions, you must rely on your physician's expertise and recommendations. It would be wonderful if everyone had unlimited time to think about their physician's recommendations, but in reality this isn't the case. If your disease or condition is a chronic, benign problem (like a plantar's wart on your foot) you may have all the time in the world to decide upon treatment. However, if you are diagnosed with an advanced malignant disease like lung cancer that has spread to other areas of the body, then you may not have much time at all to decide what to do. Or, if you have an emergency (like a heart attack) and you are in the emergency room, you may have no choice but to immediately follow the physician's recommendations.

Unless you are in an emergency situation (e.g., having a heart attack), you usually have a least a little time to decide what to do next. Always ask your physician how much time you do have to decide upon treatment. They may not have an exact answer, but they should be able to give you at least an approximate answer. This will let you know how fast you or your loved one need to investigate your treatment options including things like second or third opinions (see Chapter 5).

Collecting Your Medical Information

Collecting your patient information is something you really need to do. It's a good idea to do this for routine tests as well as difficult diagnoses. If you keep track of your own medical test results, it will be much easier for you to understand your health and be able to share this information with other health care providers as needed. Collecting your medical information means having written copies of your test results, letters, diagnoses, and treatment recommendations from your physicians. You have every right to ask for your medical information; after all — it is all about you!

You will have to work with your physician's office or medical facility to get your medical information. What this means is that you may not be able to get copies of your information immediately. Remember, your physician's office first responsibility is to provide medical care. You may have to return for your medical information. Larger offices often have staff members whose jobs are to handle medical records. If the office has a medical records person, then not just anyone can collect and copy your records for you. If you have a problem that needs immediate treatment, then you need to be persistent in getting your records as soon as possible. If you need immediate treatment, then most offices will try to help you with your records request as quickly as possible.

HIPAA

How you are able to obtain your medical information has also changed dramatically with the HIPAA laws that went into effect for health care providers on April 14, 2003. HIPAA stands for Health Insurance Portability and Accountability Act of 1996. HIPAA affects who can have your medical information and how they can use it. HIPAA limits access to your medical records to legitimate purposes such as treatment or payment and for other purposes permitted and required by law. HIPAA requires that everybody who has access to your medical records has to be able to prove they have a plan for keeping your records private. You are entitled to know each provider's (doctors, pharmacists, insurance companies, and others) plan to keep your information private. You may receive a copy of the plan or review the details. After giving you the information on how they are going to protect your privacy, then health care providers ask you to sign a form stating you have received or have had the opportunity to review their specific plan.

Although the actual HIPAA rules are very detailed, the main idea is simple: HIPAA rules give you new rights to know about — and to control — how your health information gets used. Highlights about how the HIPAA rules affect you (from www.webmd.com) can be summarized in the following ways:

❖ Your health care provider and your insurance company have to explain how they'll use and disclose health information.

❖ You can ask for copies of all this information, and make appropriate changes to it. You can also ask for a history of an unusual disclosure.

❖ If someone wants to share your health information, you have to give your formal consent.

❖ You have the right to complain to HHS (U.S. Department of Health and Human Services) about violations of HIPAA rules.

❖ Health information is to be used only for health purposes. Without your consent, it can't be used to help banks decide whether to give you a loan, or by potential employers to decide whether to give you a job.

❖ When your health information gets shared, only the minimum necessary amount of information should be disclosed.

❖ Psychotherapy records get an extra level of protection.

These new HIPAA laws may mean signing more office forms to get your medical information, or picking up your information in writing instead of over the phone. Getting your medical information is still possible; it just may take more patience on your part. However, the increased security measures resulting from the HIPAA laws have greatly changed the ability of loved ones to obtain your information. No one can obtain your medical information without your consent and without the appropriate paperwork being filled out. You will need to follow your physician's, hospital's or health care provider's office policy, but remember, in the end you are entitled to all of your medical records in writing.

Questions to Ask after the Diagnosis

Many of the important questions you need to ask about a disease or condition are listed on two forms in this section titled *Questions to Ask after the Diagnosis, Part I — Initial Questions* and *Questions to Ask after the Diagnosis, Part II — Specific Treatment Recommendations*. As their titles imply, the *Part I* form should be used when you are first diagnosed with a disease or condition, while the *Part II* form is more helpful after many initial questions have already been answered and you are trying to compare different treatment options.

Both these forms should be read before your appointment(s) with your doctor(s). They should also be taken with you to all your appointments, so you can ask the doctor or the medical staff to help fill in the form. The idea is to fill in as much information as possible on each visit. It may take several appointments to be able to fill in all the necessary answers. There is an area on each form to write in other questions that come to mind for your specific situation.

Questions to Ask after the Diagnosis
Part I — Initial Questions

This form is meant to be used when you are first diagnosed with a disease or condition, so it includes a section for *initial* treatment recommendations. Most likely you will be using this *Part I* form when discussing your problem with your primary care physician (internist, family practitioner, pediatrician, etc.) often before you see a specialist or seek additional opinions. The *Part I* form can help you understand as much as possible about your medical problem as quickly as possible. This form includes questions and issues such as:

❖ What are your main symptoms (problems)?

❖ What words describe your disease or illness?

❖ What is the name of your *suspected* disease or condition?

❖ Second/third opinion recommended?

❖ How much time do I have to make treatment decisions?

❖ Initial treatment recommendations.

❖ Additional testing needed?

❖ Additional office visits?

❖ Possible treatment options.

❖ Medications needed?

❖ Changes needed (diet, exercise, habit cessation, etc.)?

❖ Referral needed?

❖ Collecting medical information.

❖ Other questions?

With regards to collecting medical information, it is better to request copies of your test results at the office visit at which they are discussed. By doing so, you may be able to take the copies home with you the same day or at the least you will have started the process so you can obtain your copies sooner. This will help you keep your test result copies current and will prevent you from having to ask for many different test results at a later date.

An example of a completed *Part I* form can be found on the next page. (For photocopying purposes, a blank *Questions to Ask after the Diagnosis, Part I — Initial Diagnosis* form can be found in Appendix 1.)

Questions to Ask after the Diagnosis
Part I — Initial Questions *(page 1)*

Your Name: _IMA Smart Patient_

Doctor's Name: _I Can Help, M.D._

Doctor's Phone #: _313-321-3000_

Today's Date: _December 22, 2003_

1. What are your main symptoms (problems)? _Difficulty eating/_
swallowing (acid reflux), weight loss, anxiety,
heart palpations

2. Circle all words that describe your disease or illness.

    Mild   Moderate   Severe

    Acute   (Chronic)

    Benign   Malignant Not Sure Yet

    Stage I   Stage II   Stage III   Stage IV

3. What is the name of your *suspected* disease or condition? _Probably_
Hashimoto's thyroiditis; solid area found in right lobe
of thyroid gland with ultrasound test — need to rule
out cancer.

Questions to Ask after the Diagnosis
Part I — Initial Questions *(page 2)*

4. Second/third opinion recommended?

Specialist? <u>Not yet</u>

Type/whom/when? _____

Therapist (physical/ psychological/occupational, etc.)?_____

_____

Type/whom/when? _____

5. How much time do I have to make treatment decisions?

_____Days   __X__Weeks   _____Months

6. Initial treatment recommendations:

Additional testing needed (ex: blood tests, x-rays, CAT scan, MRI, biopsy, etc.)?

What test? <u>Needle biopsy of solid area found in right lobe of thyroid</u>

When? <u>ASAP</u>

What test? _____

When? _____

What test? _____

When? _____

Additional office visits?

Doctor: <u>I Can Help, M.D.</u>

When? <u>After needle biopsy — to get results of biopsy</u>

Doctor:_____

When? _____

Doctor:_____

When? _____

Questions to Ask after the Diagnosis
Part I — Initial Questions *(page 3)*

Possible treatment options:

Medication only? _____

Surgery? _May be needed to remove solid area;_
need biopsy results first

Radiation? _____

Chemotherapy? _____

Therapy (physical/ psychological/occupational, etc.)? _____

_____

Other? _____

Medications needed?

What? _Nexium®_

How much, when? _40 mg capsule taken once/day on_
empty stomach

What? _____

How much, when? _____

_____

Changes needed?

Diet? _Avoid foods that aggravate acid reflux_
(spicy, caffeine, etc.)

Exercise? _____

Habit cessation (smoking/alcohol/drugs, etc.)? _____

Other? _____

Questions to Ask after the Diagnosis
Part I — Initial Questions *(page 4)*

Note: Initial treatment recommendations should be followed with specific treatment recommendations as soon as enough information is available — see form, *Questions to Ask after the Diagnosis, Part II — Specific Treatment Recommendations.*

Referral needed?

Specialist? <u>Yes, for ultrasound guided needle biopsy</u>
<u>of thyroid</u>

Type/whom/when? <u>Radiologist/Dr. IC Well/ASAP</u>

_____

Therapist (physical/psychological/occupational, etc.)? _____

_____

Type/whom/when _____

_____

7. Collecting medical information

Do you have copies of?

_____Diagnosis   __X__Test results (Ultrasound) _____Letters

_____Treatment recommendations   __X__Other (blood tests)

8. Other questions: _____

<u>If biopsy results show a problem — who should I see next?</u>
<u>Answer: Surgeon who operates on thyroid glands</u>
<u>(endocrine surgeon)</u>
<u>Who? Dr. Steady Hands</u>

_____

Questions to Ask after the Diagnosis
Part II — Specific Treatment Recommendations

The *Part II* form should be used after you have used the form *Questions to Ask after the Diagnosis, Part I — Initial Questions*. The *Part I* form is the form you should have been using initially to gather information about your particular disease or condition. By now, it should contain important facts and history about your diagnosis.

The *Part II* form asks some of the same questions that are found in the *Part I* form, but new in-depth questions are also asked. Some of the questions need to be repeated from the *Part I* form as new information, opinions, and test results may be available. Also, another doctor may have a different opinion as to the suspected disease/condition or may need to conduct additional testing before being able to render his or her best recommendations.

After these initial similar questions, the *Part II* form then moves beyond the *Part I* form by helping you compare different specific treatment options and recommendations. These specific treatment options and recommendations may have been given to you by your current doctor or they may be the result of your seeing specialists or seeking additional opinions. The *Part II* form provides room to answer specific questions for up to three different treatment options. These treatment option questions cover areas such as:

✤ Recommended treatment(s).

✤ Length of treatment(s).

✤ Medications needed?

✤ Additional testing/monitoring?

✤ Side effects of treatment.

✤ Risks of treatment.

❖ Short and long-term prognoses (outcomes).

❖ Is the treatment covered by my insurance?

These are all very important questions/areas to think about when trying to decide which treatment option is best for you.

In addition, the *Part II* form asks other questions to help you compare care you might receive from different doctors. These questions cover areas such as:

❖ What treatment option do *you* think is in my best interest?

❖ Without any treatment, what is most likely to happen?

❖ How long will it take for these things to happen?

❖ Treatment option ___ (fill in number) was recommended to me by another doctor. Why do you think treatment option ___ (fill in number) is better?

❖ Do you offer/recommend a treatment that is unavailable elsewhere?

❖ Is there another treatment only available elsewhere for my condition?

❖ If I start treatment with you, will you follow my care or will other doctors help? How so?

❖ Who coordinates my care with other doctors and medical providers?

❖ Who do I call and how do I reach them if I have a problem during treatment?

⬦ What number do I call if I have a problem outside of regular office hours?

❖ How soon should treatment begin?

✤ Can treatment be started quickly?

✤ What do I need to do to get started?

✤ Collecting medical information.

✤ Other questions?

Although the form *Questions to Ask after the Diagnosis, Part II — Specific Treatment Recommendations* may seem long, all of the questions are important. If you do not have three treatment options recommended to you, you may not need to fill in all of the form. However, you should review the form before your appointment(s), so you can be familiar with what questions are asked and where they are located in the form.

Filling out as much of the form as applies to you is a very important step and well worth the time. After all, it is *your health at stake*. You need to make sure you are making the best possible choices. Having and understanding as much information as possible will increase your chances of making successful choices and decisions.

The *Part II* form contains questions to help you make decisions so you can help develop the best overall treatment plan for your particular problem. If you are seeing several specialists who are working together to develop a treatment plan for you, you can use the same form for more than one provider as long as space permits. However, if you are seeking additional opinions from the same type of specialists, you may want to use a new form for each of the same type of specialist you see.

An example of a completed *Part II* form can be found on pages 45–55. In this example, the same form is used for two different doctors: Dr. Thyroid Genius (endocrinologist) and Dr. Steady Hands (endocrine surgeon) because they are working together to develop treatment recommendations for IMA Smart Patient. (For photocopying purposes, a blank *Questions to Ask after the Diagnosis, Part II — Specific Treatment Recommendations* form can be found in Appendix 1.)

It is very important to get copies of all your test results and letters written by your doctors including all final information about your treatment. This important step can provide you with specific information about your test results, exact diagnoses, and treatment recommendations. You never know when you might need this information again. Having the actual test result in your medical notebook or organizer (see Chapter 5) can save you time and frustration by not having to retrieve it later from a doctor's office if you do need it again.

Questions to Ask after the Diagnosis

Part II — Specific Treatment Recommendations *(page 1)*

Your Name: _IMA Smart Patient_

Doctor's Name: _Thyroid Genius, M.D./Steady Hands, M.D._

Doctor's Specialty: _Endocrinologist/Endocrine Surgeon_

Doctor's Phone #: _734-936-4444 / 734-936-4455_

Today's Date: _February 28, 2004_

1. What are your main symptoms (problems)? _____

Difficulty eating/swallowing (acid reflux), weight loss,
anxiety, heart palpatations

_____

_____

_____

2. Circle all words that describe your disease or illness.

Mild	Moderate	Severe
Acute	(Chronic)	
Benign	Malignant	? Too Early Yet
Stage I	Stage II	Stage III Stage IV

3. What is the name of your *suspected* disease or condition? _____

Probably Hashimoto's thyroiditis with a hot nodule or
Graves disease — need more testing since needle biopsy
didn't have enough cells for a diagnosis

_____

_____

Questions to Ask after the Diagnosis
Part II — Specific Treatment Recommendations *(page 2)*

4. Additional testing needed (ex: blood tests, x-rays, CAT scan, MRI, biopsy, etc.)?

What test? <u>Blood test to check TSH and free T4 levels</u>
When? <u>ASAP</u>

What test? <u>Thyroid Uptake Study</u>
When? <u>In next few weeks</u>

What test? <u>Thyroid Scan (Pinhole)</u>
When? <u>In next few weeks</u>

5. Additional office visits?

Doctor: <u>Thyroid Genius, M.D.</u>
When? <u>After additional tests to get results</u>

Doctor: <u>Steady Hands, M.D.</u>
When? <u>After appointment with Thyroid Genius, M.D. if thyroid surgery a recommendation</u>

6. Results of additional testing?

What test? <u>Blood tests (TSH and free T4)</u>
Result? <u>TSH is too low; free T4 is too high; too much thyroid hormone in blood</u>

What test? <u>Thyroid uptake</u>
Result? <u>Depressed thyroid uptake consistent with Hashimoto's thyroiditis</u>

What test? <u>Thyroid scan (pinhole)</u>
Result? <u>Dominant "hot" (overworking) nodule in right lobe with suppression of the remaining multinodular thyroid gland; most likely not malignant</u>

7. What is the *exact* name of your disease or condition after additional testing?

<u>Hashimoto's thyroiditis with a "hot" nodule in the right lobe. In simple terms, most of the thyroid gland is working at below normal levels, but the one "hot" area is overworking causing symptoms of being hyperthyroid (too much thyroid hormone)</u>

Questions to Ask after the Diagnosis

Part II — Specific Treatment Recommendations *(page 3)*

8. How much time do I have to make treatment decisions?

_____Days   ___X___Weeks   ___X___Months

9. Specifics about your treatment option(s):

OPTION #1:

Recommended treatment: _Observe the thyroid gland every few months by ultrasound and see if the "hot" nodule will disappear on its own_

Length of treatment: _Unknown_

Medications needed?

What? _Propranolol to decrease symptoms of being hyperthyroid_

How much, when? _20mg tablet once per day_

What? _Nexium® 40mg_

How much, when? _1 capsule/day as needed for acid reflux_

What?_____

How much, when? _____

Questions to Ask after the Diagnosis
Part II — Specific Treatment Recommendations *(page 4)*

Additional testing/monitoring needed? <u>Ultrasound every 6 months;</u>
<u>blood tests to check thyroid hormone levels (TSH/free T4)</u>
<u>every 3 months or as symptoms change</u>

Side effects of treatment: <u>Side effects of propranolol; symptoms</u>
<u>(feelings) of being hyperthyroid could still continue</u>

Risks of treatment: <u>"Hot" nodule may or may not ever disappear</u>
<u>on its own/propranolol may not make all the symptoms of</u>
<u>hyperthyroidism disappear (could still feel poorly for a long time)</u>

Short-term prognosis: <u>Depends upon how much propranolol</u>
<u>decreases symptoms of hyperthyroidism</u>

Long-term prognosis: <u>Unknown since "hot" nodule may not</u>
<u>disappear on its own</u>

Is treatment covered by my insurance?

No

(Yes) – If yes, at what percentage(s)? <u>Covered at rates for office visits, testing and</u>
<u>prescriptions — better if stay in network — both of these doctors are in network</u>

Other payment questions (see *Insurance Form* in Chapter 6): _____

_____

_____

_____

Questions to Ask after the Diagnosis
Part II — Specific Treatment Recommendations *(page 5)*

OPTION #2:

Recommended treatment: <u>Surgically remove right half of thyroid gland (part</u> <u>that has "hot" nodule); replacement thyroid hormone would probably be needed</u> <u>for life since would only have 1/2 of thyroid gland remaining</u>

Length of treatment: <u>Surgery would require one- to two-day</u> <u>hospital stay; recovery from surgery about 4 weeks;</u> <u>replacement thyroid hormone (daily tablet) needed for life</u>

Medications needed?

What? <u>Levoxyl®</u>

How much, when? <u>One tablet daily, amount depends upon</u> <u>blood levels and could take 6-10 months to adjust to</u> <u>long-term dose amount</u>

What? <u>Calcium supplements</u>

How much, when? <u>May need calcium supplements daily if parathyroid</u> <u>hormones (involved in maintaining calcium levels in body) are</u> <u>disturbed during surgery; amount depends upon blood levels</u>

What? <u>Nexium® 40mg</u>

How much, when? <u>1 capsule/day as needed for acid reflux</u>

Additional testing/monitoring needed? <u>Biopsy removed thyroid</u> <u>gland to make sure nodule is not malignant; blood tests</u> <u>periodically to monitor TSH, free T4, calcium</u>

Questions to Ask after the Diagnosis
Part II — Specific Treatment Recommendations *(page 6)*

Side effects of treatment: May need to adjust dosage amounts of Levoxyl® and or calcium supplement for months

Risks of treatment: Usual surgical risks, infection, right parathyroid glands may not function, nerve affecting vocal cords could be injured and not recover; left 1/2 of thyroid gland that was not removed could develop a "hot" nodule at a later date and surgery could be required again

Short-term prognosis: Depends upon recovery from surgery

Long-term prognosis: Good if parathyroid glands function well, there is no nerve damage, and adequate Levoxyl® dose is found; if problem with any of these areas, then prognosis not as good

Is treatment covered by my insurance?

No

(Yes)- If yes, at what percentage(s)? In-network hospital costs are covered at 85% up to individual maximum of $2000/year

Other payment questions (see *Insurance Form* in Chapter 6): _____

Questions to Ask after the Diagnosis

Part II — Specific Treatment Recommendations *(page 7)*

OPTION #3:

Recommended treatment: <u>Surgically remove entire thyroid gland;</u>
<u>replacement thyroid hormone would be needed for life</u>

Length of treatment: <u>Surgery would require one- to two-day</u>
<u>hospital stay; recovery from surgery about 4 weeks;</u>
<u>replacement thyroid hormone (daily tablet) needed for life</u>

Medications needed?

What? <u>Levoxyl®</u>

How much, when? <u>One tablet daily (starting dose 125mcg),</u>
<u>amount depends upon blood levels and could take</u>
<u>6-10 months to adjust to long-term dose amount</u>

What? <u>Calcium supplements</u>

How much, when? <u>May need calcium supplements daily if parathyroid</u>
<u>hormones (involved in maintaining calcium levels in body) are</u>
<u>disturbed during surgery; amount depends upon blood levels</u>

What? <u>Nexium® 40mg</u>

How much, when? <u>1 capsule/day as needed for acid reflux</u>

Additional testing/monitoring needed? <u>Biopsy removed thyroid</u>
<u>gland to make sure nodule is not malignant; blood tests</u>
<u>periodically to monitor TSH, free T4, calcium</u>

51

Questions to Ask after the Diagnosis
Part II — Specific Treatment Recommendations *(page 8)*

Side effects of treatment: <u>May need to adjust dosage amounts</u>
<u>of Levoxyl® and or calcium supplement for months</u>

Risks of treatment: <u>Usual surgical risks, infection, all</u>
<u>parathyroid glands may not function, nerve affecting</u>
<u>vocal cords could be injured and not recover</u>

Short-term prognosis: <u>Depends upon recovery from surgery</u>

Long-term prognosis: <u>Good if parathyroid glands function well, there</u>
<u>is no nerve damage, and adequate Levoxyl® dose is found; if</u>
<u>problem with any of these areas then prognosis not as good</u>

Is treatment covered by my insurance?

  No

  (Yes)– If yes, at what percentage(s)? <u>In-network hospital costs are</u>
<u>covered at 85% up to individual maximum of $2000/year</u>

  Other payment questions (see *Insurance Form* in Chapter 6): _____

Questions to Ask after the Diagnosis

Part II — Specific Treatment Recommendations *(page 9)*

10. What treatment option do *you* think is in my best interest? Since it is unknown if the "hot" nodule will ever disappear on its own, surgery is the best long-term option. Removing the entire gland makes more sense than just removing 1/2 of the gland since no new nodules can form at a later time requiring additional surgery. This option does require thyroid replacement hormone for life and does have the surgical risks previously described

11. Without any treatment, what is most likely to happen? Symptoms of hyperthyroidism will remain as long as "hot" nodule remains. Propranolol treatment only may not eliminate the symptoms enough for you to function and feel well.

How long will it take for these things to happen? Unsure

12. Treatment option __#1__ (fill in number) was recommended to me by another doctor.

Why do you think treatment option #3 (fill in number) is better?
Already discussed in questions #10 and #11

13. Do you offer/recommend a treatment that is unavailable elsewhere?
Excellent care at a top-rated hospital in the country. Plus, as an endocrine surgeon, I do thyroid surgery hundreds of times per year.

14. Is there another treatment only available elsewhere for my condition?
No

Questions to Ask after the Diagnosis
Part II — Specific Treatment Recommendations *(page 10)*

15. If I start treatment with you, will you follow my care or will other doctors help? How so? You may see residents (doctors in training) at some points of your hospital stay, but I (Dr. Steady Hands) will be doing your surgery and I will see you each day in the hospital as well. Once you have recovered from the surgery, I will refer you back to Dr. Thyroid Genius for adjustments in your medications and periodic blood testing.

16. Who coordinates my care with other doctors and medical providers? Myself (Dr. Steady Hands) or my nurse initially, then Dr. Thyroid Genius.

17. Who do I call and how do I reach them if I have a problem during treatment? My nurse at 734-555-4477 unless it is an emergency; she will let me know what is going on. If it is an emergency (throat swelling, bleeding) you should go to the nearest hospital.

What number do I call if I have a problem outside of regular office hours? The endocrine resident on call can be reached at 734-555-4488 any time of the day or night

18. How soon should treatment begin? As soon as it can be scheduled and you are ready

Questions to Ask after the Diagnosis

Part II — Specific Treatment Recommendations *(page 11)*

19. Can treatment be started quickly? <u>Within the next few weeks</u>

_____

20. What do I need to do to get started? <u>Schedule the necessary</u> <u>surgical appointments (pre-operative appointment and</u> <u>surgery date) and speak with billing to answer any</u> <u>insurance questions you may have</u>

_____

21. Collecting medical information

I would like copies of:

___X___ Diagnosis   ___X___ Test results   ___X___ Letters

___X___ Treatment recommendations   _____ Other

22. Other questions: <u>How long have you been a surgeon?</u>
<u>Answer: 10 years</u>
<u>Since I have a latex allergy, is the hospital prepared to</u>
<u>care for people with this allergy?</u>
<u>Answer: Yes, and because of your allergy you will be</u>
<u>the first surgical case of the day (lesser chance of</u>
<u>reacting to air-borne latex).</u>

_____

_____

_____

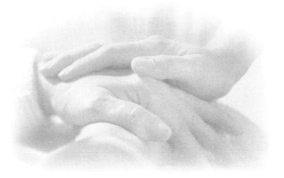

CHAPTER 3

Understanding the Basics

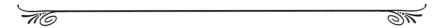

This chapter is written to help take some of the mystery out of *doctor speak*. While it is helpful to understand some basic medical terms and information, no one expects you to memorize this entire chapter. The text presented here is reference material you can come back to as you need it. You may hear many of these medical terms at your various appointments or you may read these terms in your medical records.

As you read this chapter, remember that physicians and health care workers spend years learning medical terms and information. They use these words to be able to speak with (and understand) other health care providers. You need to learn how to understand your disease or condition, not earn a medical degree. You can use this chapter to look up the words you need to know. If you can't find a word you are looking for, other reference sources such as a medical dictionary can help. Medical dictionaries are dictionaries containing medical terms and they can be found at libraries, bookstores, or on the Internet. Chapter 4 will explain more about where you can go to find out more information about your disease or condition.

This chapter will provide information about:

✤ Medical terms.

✤ Common medical tests.

✤ How to read test results.

✤ Prescription drugs.

✤ Health care provider abbreviations.

✤ Medical and dental specialists.

Medical Terms

As you begin to learn basic medical terms it is important to realize that many of them are often made up of several smaller terms. Sometimes you will find multiple medical terms listed in the dictionary in their entirety, just as you are looking for them. A good example of a medical term, which can be found in the dictionary and that's made up of several smaller words is *periapical abscess*. When this term is broken apart word by word there are three parts:

✤ peri- (around).

✤ apical (apex or end of a tooth root).

✤ abscess (infection).

So, a *periapical abscess* means an infection around the root of a tooth (*Mosby's Medical Dictionary*, 2002).

Another example is the medical term *polyarthritis*. This term is made up of the following three parts:

❖ poly (many).

❖ arthro- (joint).

❖ -itis (inflammation).

So, *polyarthritis* means inflammation of more than one joint (*Mosby's Medical Dictionary*, 2002).

Sometimes you may not find a grouping of medical terms listed in their entirety in the dictionary under one entry. Instead, you may have to look up several medical terms and then combine the meanings. It's not unusual to find several medical terms combined together to describe a tumor found during a test or biopsy. The terms used can be used to describe where and what the tumor is. An example of this is a biopsy description of a *2.4cm, invasive squamous cell carcinoma within the right bronchus intermedius*. The description can be broken down word by word as follows (*Mosby's Medical Dictionary*, 2002):

❖ 2.4cm (size of the biopsy).

❖ invasive (spreading or invading).

❖ squamous cell (a flat cell usually covering another tissue).

❖ carcinoma (cancer).

❖ bronchus (any one of several large air passages/branches in the lungs through which inhaled air and exhaled air pass).

❖ intermedius (an element between structures, *Stedman's Medical Dictionary*, 1982).

Therefore, a biopsy description of a *2.4cm, invasive squamous cell carcinoma within the right bronchus intermedius* means a 2.4cm, invading squamous cell malignant tumor was found inside the right lung between two bronchus (passageways). In simplest terms, the description means that lung cancer was found in the lining of the air passages leading to part of the right lung and it was spreading or invading. It was located between two passageways and it was made up of cells called squamous epithelium cells. This biopsy found a serious malignant tumor that was spreading. All of the words used to describe the tumor were important because they tell more and more information about the tumor. The size of the tumor, the type of tumor cells found, where they are found, and if they are invading are all important facts in helping to determine the right treatment. While you would never find all these words together in the dictionary under one entry, all of these words and/or phrases can be found separately in a medical dictionary, and when the meanings are put together they can provide a great deal of information.

In the beginning, having to combine words or look up multiple words can seem daunting, but have patience and take it one word at a time. You can do it.

Table 1 lists some of the more commonly used medical terms. The chart has a column of official definitions as well as a column of words to think of for each medical term. Sometimes it is easier to learn medical terms by thinking of a few key words at first. The definitions are all from *Mosby's Medical Dictionary* (2002) unless otherwise noted.

Commonly Used Medical Terms

Table 1

WORD	DEFINITION	THINK
Abscess	A cavity containing pus and surrounded by inflamed tissue.	Pocket of pus
Acute	(Of a disease or disease symptoms) beginning abruptly with marked intensity or sharpness, then subsiding after a relatively short period.	Short or new problem, painful illness
Allergy	A hypersensitive reaction to common, often intrinsically harmless, substances most of which are environmental. Symptoms of mild allergies, such as those associated with rhinitis, conjunctivitis and urticaria, can be suppressed by antihistamines with glucocorticoids administered as supplements to primary therapy. Severe allergic reactions, such as anaphylaxis and angioneurotic edema of the glottis, can cause systemic shock and death and commonly require immediate therapy with subcutaneous epinephrine or IV steroids.	Mild allergy— watery eyes, runny nose and itching

Severge allergy— whole body reaction or trouble breathing (Can cause death) |
| Anorexia | Lack or loss of appetite, resulting in the inability to eat. | Eating disorder making people too thin |
| Anti- | Prefix meaning against or over against. | Against |

WORD	DEFINITION	THINK
Antibiotic	Pertaining to the ability to destroy or interfere with a living organism. An antimicrobial agent, derived from cultures of a microorganism or produced semisynthetically, used to treat infections.	Medicine to fight infections caused by bacteria
Antihistamine	Any substance capable of reducing the physiologic and pharmacologic effects of histamine, including a wide variety of drugs that block histamine receptors. Many such drugs are available as nonprescription drugs for the management of allergies.	Allergy medicine
Antiviral	Destructive to viruses.	Medicine to fight infections caused by a virus
Apical	Pertaining to the summit or apex, pertaining to the end of a tooth root.	The top, the end, or the summit of a structure.
Artery	One of the large blood vessels carrying blood in a direction away from the heart to the tissues.	Blood vessel carrying oxygen rich blood
Arthritis	Any inflammatory condition of the joints, characterized by pain, swelling, heat, redness, and limitation of movement.	Painful inflammation of the joints

WORD	DEFINITION	THINK
Asthma	A respiratory disorder characterized by recurring episodes of paroxysmal dyspnea, wheezing on expiration and/or inspiration caused by constriction of the bronchi, coughing, and viscous mucoid bronchial secretions.	Illness that causes difficulty breathing including wheezing
Benign	(Of a tumor) noncancerous and therefore not an immediate threat, even though treatment eventually may be required for health or cosmetic reasons.	Noncancerous tumor
Biopsy	The removal of a small piece of living tissue from an organ or other part of the body for microscopic examination to confirm or establish a diagnosis, estimate prognosis, or follow the course of a disease.	Removal of tissue for microscopic examination
Bulimia	A disorder characterized by an insatiable craving for food, often resulting in episodes of continuous eating and often followed by purging, depression, and self-deprivation.	Eating disorder involving binging and purging
CA 125	Abbreviation for cancer cell surface antigen 125. The CA 125 tumor marker test is a blood test used to detect ovarian cancer and to monitor the patient's response to therapy.	Blood test to detect ovarian cancer

WORD	DEFINITION	THINK
Calorie	A unit equal to the large calorie, used to denote the heat expenditure of an organism and the fuel or energy valued of food.	Food energy counted by dieters, dieticians, etc.
Cancer	A neoplasm characterized by the uncontrolled growth of anaplastic cells that tend to invade surrounding tissue and to metastasize to distant body sites.	Cancerous tumor — fast growing cells that can kill a person
Cancer staging	A system for describing the size and extent of spread of a malignant tumor, used to plan treatment and predict prognosis. Staging may involve a physical examination, diagnostic procedures, surgical exploration and histological examination. The system developed by the American Joint Committee for Cancer Staging and End Results Reporting uses the letter T to represent the tumor, N for the regional lymph node involvement, M for distant metastases, and numeric subscripts in each category to indicate the degree of dissemination.	**TNM** **T** is for tumor **N** is for lymph node involvement **M** is for metastases
Carbohydrate	Any of a group of organic compounds, the most important of which are the saccharides, starch, cellulose, and glycogen.	Compounds found in foods counted by dieters, dieticians, etc.

WORD	DEFINITION	THINK
Cardiovascular	Pertaining to the heart and blood vessels.	Heart and blood vessels
Cataract	An abnormal progressive condition of the lens of the eye, characterized by loss of transparency.	Clouding of the eye lens
Catheter	A hollow flexible tube that can be inserted into a vessel or cavity of the body to withdraw or to instill fluids, directly monitor various types of information, and visualize a vessel or cavity.	Hollow flexible tube
Central	Pertaining to or situated at a center.	Center
Cholesterol	A waxy soluble compound found only in animal tissues. A member of a group of compounds called sterols, it is an integral component of every cell in the body. Cholesterol is found in foods of animal origin and is continuously synthesized tin the body, primarily in the liver.	Compound found in animal cells (too much can increase chances for heart attack and stroke)
Chronic	(Of a disease or disorder) persisting for a long period, often for the remainder of a person's lifetime.	Long-term illness or disease
Condition	A state of being, specifically in reference to physical and mental health or well-being.	State of physical or mental being

WORD	DEFINITION	THINK
Conjunctivitis	Inflammation of the conjunctiva, caused by bacterial or viral infection, allergy or environmental factors. Red eyes, thick discharge, sticky eyelids in the morning, and inflammation without pain are characteristic results of the most common cause, bacteria.	Eye infection ("pink eye")
Contra-	Prefix meaning against.	Against
Cutaneous	Pertaining to the skin.	Skin
Cyst	An uninflammed closed sac in or under the skin lined with epithelium and containing fluid or semisolid material.	An enclosed fluid filled lump
Decongestant	Pertaining to a substance or procedure that eliminates or reduces congestion or swelling.	Medicine to reduce congestion (nasal)
Deep	Profundus, situated at a deeper level in relation to a specific reference point; opposite of superficial. *(Stedman's Medical Dictionary,* 1982)	Deep
Diabetes	A clinical condition characterized by the excessive excretion of urine. The excess may be caused by a deficiency of antidiuretic hormone (ADH), as in diabetes insipidus, or it may be the polyuria resulting from the hyperglycemia that occurs in diabetes mellitus.	If diabetes insipidus, then characterized by: Excessive urine Excessive thirst If diabetes mellitus, then characterized by: Excessive urine Excessive thirst Excessive hunger

WORD	DEFINITION	THINK
Diagnosis	Identification of a disease or condition by a scientific evaluation of physical signs, symptoms, history, laboratory test results, and procedures.	Identification of a disease or condition
Disease	A condition of abnormal vital function involving any structure, part, or system of an organism. A specific illness or disorder characterized by a recognizable set of signs and symptoms, attributable to heredity, infection, diet, or environment.	Known medical illness
Dys-	Prefix meaning bad, painful, or disordered.	Bad
Dyslexia	An impairment of the ability to read, as a result of a variety of pathologic conditions, some of which are associated with the central nervous system. Dyslexic persons often reverse letters and words, cannot adequately distinguish the letter sequences in written words, and have difficulty determining left from right.	Problem reading due to difficulties with recognizing letters and word orders
Dyspepsia	A vague feeling of epigastric discomfort after eating.	Upset stomach
Dysphagia	Difficulty in swallowing commonly associated with obstructive or motor disorders of the esophagus.	Difficulty swallowing

WORD	DEFINITION	THINK
Dyspnea	A distressful sensation of uncomfortable breathing that may be caused by certain heart conditions, strenuous exercise, or anxiety.	Difficulty breathing
Emphysema	An abnormal condition of the pulmonary system, characterized by overinflation and destructive changes in alveolar walls. It results in a loss of lung elasticity and decreased gas exchange.	Lung condition making breathing more difficult Cigarette smoking causes chronic emphysema
Front-	Combining form meaning forehead or front.	Front
Hemoglobin	A complex protein-iron compound in the blood that carries oxygen to the cells from the lungs and carbon dioxide away from the cells to the lungs.	Protein compound in blood that carries oxygen or carbon dioxide
Hyper-	Prefix meaning excessive, above, or beyond.	Excess or too much
Hyperglycemia	A greater than normal amount of glucose in the blood. Most frequently associated with diabetes mellitus.	Too much sugar in the blood
Hyperinsulinemia	An excessive amount of insulin in the body.	Too much insulin in the blood
Hypertension	A common disorder characterized by elevated blood pressure persistently exceeding 140/90 mm Hg.	High blood pressure

WORD	DEFINITION	THINK
Hyperthyroidism	A condition characterized by hyperactivity of the thyroid gland.	Too much thyroid hormone
Hypo-	Prefix meaning under, below, beneath, deficient or lacking oxygen.	Below or too little
Hypocalcemia	A deficiency of calcium in the serum (blood).	Too little calcium in the blood
Hypotension	An abnormal condition in which the blood pressure is not adequate for normal perfusion and oxygenation of the tissues.	Low blood pressure
Hypothyroidism	A condition characterized by decreased activity of the thyroid gland.	Too little thyroid hormone
Hysterectomy	Surgical removal of the uterus.	Removal of the uterus
Infra-	Prefix meaning situated, formed, or occurring beneath.	Beneath
Inter-	Prefix meaning situated, formed, or occurring between.	Between
Intra-	Prefix meaning situated, formed, or occurring within.	Within
Ipsi	Prefix meaning the same or self.	Same
Invasive	Characterized by a tendency to spread, infiltrate, and intrude.	Spreading, invading

WORD	DEFINITION	THINK
Lateral	Pertaining to the side, away from the midsagital plane.	Side, not central
Lipid	Any of a structurally diverse group of compounds that are insoluble in water but soluble in alcohol, chloroform, ether, and other solvents. Some lipids are stored in the body and serve as an energy reserve, but are elevated in various diseases such as atherosclerosis. Kinds of lipids include cholesterol, fatty acids, phospholipids, and triglycerides.	Fats (too much can cause heart attack and stroke)
Local	Pertaining to a small circumscribed area of the body, pertaining to a treatment or drug applied locally.	Small area of the body
Lymph	A thin, watery fluid originating in organs and tissues of the body that circulates through the lymphatic vessels and is filtered by the lymph nodes. Lymph enters the bloodstream at the junction of the internal jugular and subclavian veins. Lymph contains chyle, erythyrocytes, and leukocytes, most of which are lymphocytes.	Fluid from organs and tissues that is filtered by lymph nodes and ends up back in the bloodstream
Lymph node	One of the many small oval structures that filter the lymph and fight infection and in which lymphocytes, monocytes, and plasma cells are formed.	"Glands" (like those which swell in the neck when sick); filter lymph fluid and help fight infections

WORD	DEFINITION	THINK
Malignant	Tending to become worse and to cause death, (describing a cancer) anaplastic, invasive, and metastatic.	Cancerous, can cause death
Medial	Pertaining to, situated in, or orientated toward the midline of the body.	Near the midline of the body
Metastasis	The process by which tumor cells spread to distant parts of the body.	When tumor cells spread far from where they started
Mild	Gentle, subtle, or of low intensity, such as a mild infection.	Low or non-serious
Moderate	Tending toward the mean or average amount of dimension. (*Merriam-Webster's Collegiate Dictionary,* 2004)	Average
Musculoskeletal	Pertaining to the muscles and the skeleton.	Muscles and bones
Neoplasm	Any abnormal growth of new tissue, benign or malignant. Also called tumor.	Tumor, can be benign (non-cancerous) or malignant (cancer)
Obese	Pertaining to a corpulent or excessively heavy individual. Generally a person is regarded as medically obese if he or she is 20% above desirable body weight for the person's age, sex, height, and body build.	Carrying way too much extra weight

WORD	DEFINITION	THINK
Pap smear	A simple smear method of examining stained exfoliative cells. It is used most commonly to detect cancers of the cervix, but it may be used for tissue specimens from any organ.	Test to detect cancer of the cervix in women
Para-	Prefix meaning similar, beside, beyond, supplementary to, disordered.	Beside
Per-	Prefix meaning throughout or completely.	Throughout
Peri-	Prefix meaning around.	Around
Peripheral	Pertaining to the outside, surface, or surrounding area of an organ, other structure, or field of vision.	Outside
Pneumonia	An acute inflammation of the lungs, often caused by inhaled pneumonococci of the species *Streptococcus pneumoniae.*	Lung infection
Poly-	Prefix meaning many or much.	Many
Polydipsia	Excessive thirst.	Too thirsty
Polyphagia	Excessive uncontrolled eating.	Too much eating
Polyuria	The excretion of an abnormally large amount of urine.	Too much urine
Prognosis	A prediction of the probable outcome of a disease based on the condition of the person and usual course of the disease as observed in similar situations.	Probable disease outcome

WORD	DEFINITION	THINK
Proximal	Nearer to a point of reference or attachment, usually the trunk of the body, than other parts of the body.	Nearer Often the trunk of the body
PSA	Abbreviation for prostate-specific antigen. The PSA test is a blood test used to detect prostatic cancer and to monitor the patient's response to therapy.	Blood test to detect prostate cancer
Pulmonary	Pertaining to the lungs or the respiratory system.	Lung
Rejection	An immunologic attack against organ or substances that the immune system recognizes as foreign, including grafts and transplants.	Body attacking a graft or transplant
Retro-	Prefix meaning backward or located behind.	Backward or located behind
Rhinitis	Inflammation of the mucous membranes of the nose, usually accompanied by swelling of the mucosa and a nasal discharge.	Congested, drippy nose
Severe	Of a great degree or serious. (*Merriam-Webster's Collegiate Dictionary*, 2004)	High or serious
Stage	A period or phase.	Period or phase
Staging	The classification of phases or period of a disease or other pathologic process, as in the TNM clinical method of assigning numerical values to various stages of tumor development.	Figuring out how far along a disease is (**T** is for tumor **N** is for lymph node involvement **M** is for metastases)

WORD	DEFINITION	THINK
Subacute	Less than acute, pertaining to a disease or other abnormal condition present in a person who appears to be clinically well. The condition may be identified or discovered by means of a laboratory test or radiologic examination.	Less than acute; mild, can be long-lasting
Superficial	Pertaining to the surface, not grave or dangerous.	Surface or not dangerous
Supra-	Prefix meaning above or over.	Over
Systemic	Pertaining to the whole body rather than a localized area or regional part of the body.	Involving the whole body
Terminal	(Of a structure or process) near or approaching its end, such as a terminal bronchiole or a terminal disease.	End Often used to describe a terminal illness, an illness that will cause someone to die
TNM	A system for staging malignant neoplastic disease. See also Cancer staging.	**T** is for tumor **N** is for lymph node **M** is for metastases
Topical	Pertaining to the surface of a part of the body, to a drug or treatment applied topically.	Surface or applied to the surface
Transplant	To transfer an organ or tissue from one person to another or from one body part to another to replace a disease structure, restore function, or change appearance.	Transfer an organ or tissue

WORD	DEFINITION	THINK
Tumor	A swelling or enlargement occurring in inflammatory conditions. Also called neoplasm. A new growth of tissue characterized by progressive, uncontrolled proliferation of cells.	A lump or growth, can be benign (non-cancerous) or malignant (cancer)
Urticaria	A pruritic skin eruption characterized by transient wheals of varying shapes and size with well-defined erythmatous margins and pale centers.	Hives
Vein	Any one of the many vessels that convey blood from the capillaries as part of the pulmonary venous system, the systemic venous network, or the portal venous complex (back to the heart).	Blood vessel carrying blood back to the heart

Common Medical Tests

Above and beyond medical terms, it is important to understand the common medical tests you may be asked to undergo. Your doctor, doctor's staff, or someone at the testing site you are going to should be able to explain the test and what you can expect to happen. It's best if they explain it to you because they know your medical history, current medications, and any health problems you may be experiencing.

If you are not offered written instructions about your specific test, you can still find out about the medical test you are being asked to

> *It's always a good idea to ask if your doctor's office or the testing site has written instructions about the test you are being asked to take. It is much easier to follow written instructions than to try and remember everything said during a conversation.*

take. If you have access to the Internet, you can find information about medical tests from medical websites (see Chapter 4 for a list of websites).

There are also many books that describe medical tests. Some of the books are detailed and technical sounding (i.e., *Mosby's Manual of Diagnostic and Laboratory Tests*, 2002), while other books can be easily read by someone not in the medical field (i.e., *The Encyclopedia of Medical Tests*, 1997). Your local bookstore clerk or librarian should be able to help you find a book that is right for you. If you will be undergoing many medical tests you might want to consider buying a book about them. It can be a great reference tool to have at your finger-tips when you need it. Combining information from more than one reference site (books, web-sites, etc.) can also help you understand a test much better.

Regardless of what medical test you are taking and how you are getting all of your information about it, you need basic questions answered. Specifically, you need to know the answer to the following four questions:

1. Why is the test being done?

2. What preparation is needed? Make sure you know before you have a test taken. Asking this question before the test might save you from having to go back again another day.

Examples of some preparations may include: adjusting your medications, fasting (not eating for a period of time), or taking a medication a set number of hours before a test.

3. How is the test taken?

4. Once the test is over, what, if any, aftercare is needed?

No matter what test you are undergoing, it's important to be sure that your doctor and the health care providers giving the test know your medical history and what medications you are taking. Some medications may interfere with the test results or may cause problems after the test. As an example, patients who take blood thinners may have more bleeding after a blood test. More pressure on the spot where the blood was drawn might be needed than for someone who doesn't take blood thinners. It is up to your doctor and health care providers to decide if any of your medications need to be adjusted before you take a medical test. It's your responsibility to ask and help remind them of what medications you are taking.

The remainder of this chapter will describe some of the more common medical tests you may be asked to go through. Although a brief description is provided, you should still ask your doctor's office or the testing site you plan to attend the four questions listed above for your specific medical test.

Angiogram (Arteriogram)

An angiogram is an x-ray taken of a blood vessel after injection of a radiopaque contrast medium which makes the blood vessel visible. Angiograms are usually carried out in a special procedure room with surgical and x-ray equipment. The patient lies flat and still on an examination table. After locally numbing the skin over an artery, a needle or catheter (hollow flexible tube) is placed into the artery and a contrast dye is injected into the artery. Some people will feel warm, flushed, nauseated, or have a metallic or salty taste in their mouth from the contrast dye. X-rays are taken during the injection and afterwards as well. After the test the patient is usually kept on bed rest for several hours and watched carefully. The circulation of any area of the body can be studied, but common tests include carotid angiogram (neck), cerebral angiogram (brain), and the coronary angiogram (blood vessels of the heart) (*The Encyclopedia of Medical Tests*, 1997).

Biopsy

A biopsy is a form of surgery performed to remove tissue for laboratory examination (*The Encyclopedia of Medical Tests*, 1997). A biopsy can be done on any organ as long as the area in question can be reached through surgery and removing part of the area will not cause more damage. Sometimes a biopsy removes a piece of the area in question (i.e., lung). Sometimes a biopsy removes the entire area in question (i.e., skin). And sometimes only cells and fluid are removed during the biopsy (i.e., needle biopsy of the thyroid or breast). Skin biopsies can usually be done in a doctor's office, while biopsies of other areas (like lung) may be outpatient procedures or require hospitalization. Biopsies are usually done to help make a specific diagnosis or to rule out cancer.

Blood Tests

There are numerous blood tests that can be run from a patient's blood. It's up to your doctor or health care provider to determine which blood test(s) you may need. Most blood tests are taken by drawing blood from a vein (usually in the crook of your elbow) using a needle. The needle is inserted into the vein after placing a tourniquet on the upper arm, cleaning off the site with an antiseptic, usually alcohol, and asking the patient to make a fist. The tourniquet is released and enough blood is withdrawn for testing. After the needle is removed, gauze or a cotton ball is placed over the site and slight pressure should be put on the site to help stop any bleeding. Elevating the arm can also help reduce the bleeding. A band-aid or gauze is then placed over the site (*Mosby's Manual of Diagnostic and Laboratory Test*, 2002).

CAT Scan or CT (Computerized Axial Tomography or Computed Tomography)

A CT scan is an x-ray test which can show the internal organs. The images are constructed from multiple radiation readings. Any part of the body may be scanned, such as the abdomen, joints, bones, head, larynx, eye socket, sinuses, pelvis, spine, and chest. A CT scan is good for detecting brain tumors and other diseases within the skull and for evaluating chest and abdominal cancers and injuries. It can also be used to guide instruments during a biopsy and to plan surgeries. The patient lies on a table while the CT scanner revolves around the table taking x-rays. The machine makes clicking and whirring noises as it operates. The test can be done with or without a contrast dye. A computer is used to translate the hundreds of thousands x-ray readings into multiple cross sectional images (*The Encyclopedia of Medical Tests*, 1997).

Electrocardiogram (EKG or ECG)

An EKG test measures the electrical activity of the heart and it is the most common test of heart function. For this test, multiple electrodes are attached to the chest (sometimes the ankles and wrists too) with an adhesive gel, and they record the electrical impulses. Sometimes the test is run quickly by itself or as an aid to help other tests such as a stress test or a Holter monitor (EKGs taken over 24 hours or more). An EKG test is often given when a patient has chest pain, shortness of breath, palpitations, and other symptoms suspicious for heart disease. The EKG test is based on the idea that the electrical activity of the heart can be recorded as characteristic patterns, which changes with heart disease. Characteristic patterns can be seen with recent and ongoing heart attacks, old heart attacks, heart enlargement, pericarditis, ventricular aneurysms, conduction defects, and the effects of drugs and electrolytes (*The Encyclopedia of Medical Tests*, 1997).

Electroencephalogram (EEG)

An EEG test records brain activity. The activity is seen as waves called alpha, beta, delta, and theta. To measure brain waves, electrodes are placed on various areas of the patient's head and they record the results. The patient may be asked to remain quiet or perform different activities during the test, such as opening or closing the eyes, breathing at different rates, etc. (*Mosby's Medical Dictionary*, 2002). The test is used to diagnose problems like epilepsy, meningitis, encephalitis, head injuries, strokes, brain abscesses, and brain tumors (*The Encyclopedia of Medical Tests*, 1997).

Electromyogram (EMG)

The EMG test records electrical activity in skeletal muscles. It is performed by applying surface electrodes (on the skin) or by inserting a needle electrode into the muscle and observing electrical activity (*Mosby's Medical Dictionary*, 2002). The needle is attached to an amplifier, which translates the impulses into sound and waves. The test can be uncomfortable because unfortunately no anesthesia or sedation can be given. The test is used to help diagnosis different muscle and nerve diseases (*The Encyclopedia of Medical Tests*, 1997).

Exploratory Surgery

Exploratory surgery is a surgery or operation to find the cause of a disorder by opening a body cavity or organ and examining the interior (*Mosby's Medical Dictionary*, 2002).

Laparoscopic Surgery (Laparscopy)

Laparoscopic surgery is a surgery or procedure performed with the help of an endoscope. An endoscope is "an illuminated optic instrument for visualization of the interior of a body cavity or organ" (*Mosby's Medical Dictionary*, 2002). The test is performed in a procedure room and involves either local anesthetic or general anesthetic. Carbon dioxide gas is often pumped into the abdomen before the laparoscope (endoscope) is inserted. Laparoscopy can help evaluate abdominal symptoms, fluid build-up (ascites), liver disease, cancer, and gynecological diseases. Surgical procedures such as biopsies, cultures, cauterizations, tubal ligation, and gall bladder surgeries can be performed (*The Encyclopedia of Medical Tests*, 1997).

MRI (Magnetic Resonance Imaging)

An MRI test is a medical imaging test that does not use x-rays. MRI works by using an intense magnetic field. An MRI can be done on any area of the body such as the abdomen, chest, skull, bones, or heart. However, it is most valuable in producing clear views of the brain and spinal cord. MRI can produce three-dimensional images as well as cross-sectional images like CAT scans. It's better at identifying soft-tissue structures than a CAT scan. However, since metal reacts unfavorably during the MRI, patients who have metal within their body (pacemakers, metallic aneurysm clips, some metallic prostheses, and foreign objects) cannot have this test done. During an MRI a computer turns the magnetic field on and off very rapidly. The magnetic field is so strong it causes hydrogen atoms to line up all in the same direction. When it is switched off, the hydrogen atoms "relax" to their previous direction. When the atoms relax, they give off their own magnetic field which the computer senses, reads, and processes into images. When an MRI is performed the patient is placed in an enclosed structure. Although the test is painless, there are loud noises that occur during the test and patients that suffer from claustrophobia may need to be sedated (*The Encyclopedia of Medical Tests*, 1997). An MRI may be performed with contrast dye as well.

Pap Smear (Papanicolaous's Test or Pap Test)

A Pap smear is a simple smear method of examining stained exfoliative (cells obtained by scraping or smearing) cells. The test is named after a Greek physician who practiced in the United States (George N. Papanicolaou, M.D.). The test can be used for tissue specimens from any organ, but it is used most commonly to detect cancers of the female cervix (*Mosby's Medical Dictionary*, 2002). A Pap smear is usually performed as a routine part of a pelvic examination for women. In addition to identifying cancers and precancerous conditions of the cervix, it can also help detect certain vaginal infections (*The Encyclopedia of Medical Tests*, 1997).

PET Scan (Positron Emission Tomography)

A PET scan is a computerized radiographic test that uses radioactive substances to examine the metabolic activity of various body structures, especially the brain. The patient either inhales or is injected with a metabolically important substance such as glucose (sugar) that is labeled with a radioactive element that emits positrons. When the positrons combine with electrons normally found in the cells of the body, gamma rays are emitted. The gamma rays are measured and a computer constructs color-coded images that indicate the amount of metabolic activity throughout the organ involved. PET scans are used to examine blood flow and the metabolism of the heart and blood vessels, study and diagnosis cancer, and investigate the biochemical activity of the brain (*Mosby's Medical Dictionary*, 2002).

PSA test (Prostate-Specific Antigen Test)

The PSA test is a blood test used to detect prostate cancer (in men) and to monitor the patient's response to therapy. Currently, PSA is considered the most sensitive tumor marker for this type of cancer (*Mosby's Medical Dictionary*, 2002).

Radiograph (X-Ray)

A radiograph is the image produced by x-rays. A radiograph can be taken on any area of the body and it is often used to diagnosis broken bones, joint problems, tumors, infections, and many other diseases. Radiographs are generated by x-ray machines using x-rays and special photographic film. An x-ray is an invisible ray of energy that can penetrate the body and is absorbed differently by different body structures. Structures like bone that are good at absorbing x-ray show up white on the x-ray film, while air and water absorb little x-rays, so they show up darker on the x-ray film. Internal organs like the heart and liver moderately absorb x-rays, so they show up on the x-ray film as different shades of gray (*The Encyclopedia of Medical Tests*, 1997). Since there is radiation involved with x-rays, they should be taken only if absolutely necessary on pregnant women.

Ultrasound

An ultrasound test uses sound waves to take pictures of internal organs. It can be used for almost any area of the body, including chest, abdomen, pelvis, neck, breast, extremities, eye, or penis. However, it is commonly known for its use during pregnancy. It's not normally used for the brain. While ultrasound images are not as clear as those for other imaging techniques like CAT or MRI, ultrasound remains a helpful diagnostic tool. For most areas of the body, a gel is placed on the patient's skin and then a transducer is touched to the skin to send the sound waves and record the sound waves as they bounce back from different structures. A computer helps to record the images. Ultrasound testing is painless (*The Encyclopedia of Medical Tests*, 1997).

Urinalysis

A urinalysis is a test for urine that involves a physical, microscopic, or chemical examination of urine. The specimen is physically examined for color, turbidity (how light scatters through a liquid, clear vs. cloudy), and specific gravity. The specimen is examined microscopically for blood cells, casts, crystals, pus, and bacteria. Finally the specimen is examined chemically for pH and to identify and measure levels of ketones, sugar, protein, blood components, and many other substances (*Mosby's Medical Dictionary*, 2002). A urinalysis is a common test performed and its results can help diagnose a number of conditions or diseases. Sometimes the patient may be given instructions on how to collect the urine in a certain way (clean catch technique).

Hopefully, these brief descriptions give you an idea of what these common tests involve. More detailed information on these tests and many others are available on medical websites and in books about medical testing available at your local library or bookstore.

How to Read Test Results

It is one thing to have your test results in writing, but what good is it if you cannot read them? When medical tests are taken, the results are recorded and reported so other health care providers can understand them. While there are many different possible tests that can be taken, the reported results often contain similar information. Some of the information is easy to understand, like names and dates, while other information takes more time and effort to understand. Information you might see on your test results include:

✣ Patient name (your name).

✣ Patient age (your age).

✣ Gender (your sex).

✣ Date and time of test.

✣ Type of test given (blood, EKG, CAT scan, MRI, urine, biopsy, etc.).

✣ Size of problem area or tumor.

✣ Location of problem area or tumor.

✣ Results (compared to normal findings).

✣ Diagnosis or clinical impression (can have more than one).

✣ Recommendations.

While this list can be overwhelming at first, don't panic, but try to understand one part of the report at a time. In order to read test results you must first have a copy of the results. It's a good idea to have two copies of your results so you can write on one copy and keep one copy as an original. Don't write on the original results. Having a second copy will allow you to make notes so you can better understand the report. These notes may be explanations from your doctor or from your own research or both.

It is also important to have actual copies of test results in case you need to share them with other doctors and health care providers. It is often much quicker and easier for you to provide this information than to have to wait for one doctor's office to get the information to another doctor's office.

When you speak with your doctor, get as much information about your actual results immediately. Request two copies of the results so you can keep one and write on one. If time doesn't allow this until after you see the doctor, then pay close attention to what the doctor says and ask him or her to explain the test results to you. You don't need to understand every word of the results, but you should understand the important things. Ask your doctor to explain any abnormal or unusual findings. As soon as you have two copies of the test results, write your doctor's comments on one of the copies.

Different test results will be shown on the next several pages. The results shown will be from a blood sample, a urine sample, an MRI test, and a biopsy sample. The results for each will be shown first followed by test results with notes added. This should help you understand how to read the test results. While the test results are real, names and ages have been changed to protect the privacy of the patients and doctors.

> *Note: These examples are simply that; examples. They are meant to show you how you can begin to look at important areas of test results. Specific information from these examples should not be applied to your own test results or medical conditions. Your own medical tests and conditions need to be evaluated and discussed with your medical care professionals.*

CASE STUDY

Blood Test

The first test results are for Sally Tired. Sally went to her doctor because she is always (you guessed it!) tired and she has recently gained over twenty pounds. Her doctor sent her to have blood tests run in order to check that her thyroid gland is working properly. Sally's test results are shown on the next two pages. The first page shows her original results as obtained from her doctor, while the second page has notes added to explain her results.

After getting an overall feeling for where everything is on the page, the main thing you need to do is look for any results that are abnormal or out of the normal range. Normal results should fall in between the numbers listed under normal range. In Sally's case, there are three test results out of normal range: TSH, T4, and Thyroid antibodies. Some test results are also not reported yet. You can tell this because of the words pending next to the tests for T3 and T7. So, for now, the important thing is to find out what the abnormal results for these three tests mean. Ask your doctor first! He or she should be able to explain to you in plain English what these results mean. Write down what he or she says.

Regarding Sally, her thyroid isn't working right anymore. It's not producing enough thyroid hormone (low free T4) even though the

ACCURATE LABORATORY
123 LAB STREET
ANYTOWN, USA 12345
(123) 456-7899

DR. LAB BOSS, M.D.

PATIENT NAME: SALLY TIRED
PATIENT AGE: 30
PATIENT SEX: F

DR. I CAN HELP
333 COMFORT LANE
HOMETOWN, MI 12345

PATIENT I.D. NO.   123456789
TIME OF REPORT   6:02AM
DATE OF REPORT   8/11/03
DATE OF SPECIMEN 8/9/03
DATE RECEIVED   8/9/03
TIME COLLECTED   12:00PM

TEST NAME	REFERENCE RANGE	RESULT	ABNORMAL	UNITS
THROID PROFILE				
T3 UPTAKE	PENDING			
FTI (T7)	PENDING			
THRYOID STIMULATING HORMONE (TSH)	0.29-5.11		39.91 H	IU/mL
T4, FREE	0.8-2.0		0.7 L	ng/dL
THRYOID ANTIBODIES				
THYROID MICROSOMAL AB			263.5 H	U/mL
INTERPRETATIVE DATA:				
<0.3: NON-REACTIVE				
0.3-1.0: INDETERMINATE				
>1.0: REACTIVE				
CONFIRMED IN DUPLICATE				
THYROGLOBULIN ANTIBODIES	<1.0	<1.0		u/mL

ACCURATE LABORATORY
123 LAB STREET
ANYTOWN, USA 12345
(123) 456-7899

DR. LAB BOSS, M.D.

PATIENT NAME: SALLY TIRED
PATIENT AGE: 30
PATIENT SEX: F

DR. I CAN HELP
333 COMFORT LANE
HOMETOWN, MI 12345

PATIENT I.D. NO.   123456789
TIME OF REPORT   6:02AM
DATE OF REPORT   8/11/03
DATE OF SPECIMEN   8/9/03
DATE RECEIVED   8/9/03
TIME COLLECTED   12:00PM

TEST NAME	REFERENCE RANGE	RESULT	ABNORMAL	UNITS
THROID PROFILE				
T3 UPTAKE	PENDING			
FTI (T7)	PENDING			
THRYOID STIMULATING HORMONE (TSH)	0.29-5.11		39.91 H	IU/mL
T4, FREE	0.8-2.0		0.7 L	ng/dL
THRYOID ANTIBODIES THYROID MICROSOMAL AB			263.5 H	U/mL

INTERPRETATIVE DATA:
<0.3:   NON-REACTIVE
0.3-1.0:   INDETERMINATE
>1.0:   REACTIVE

| CONFIRMED IN DUPLICATE THYROGLOBULIN ANTIBODIES | <1.0 | <1.0 | | u/mL |

(handwritten annotation, circled, pointing to PENDING) Test results are Not ready yet.

(handwritten annotation, circled, pointing to ABNORMAL values) Thyroid test results are out of normal ranges.

(handwritten annotation at bottom left)
TSH—released by pituitary gland
TSH -controls how much thyroid hormone (T4) gets released by thyroid gland
High TSH and low T4 means thyroid gland isn't working like it should (hypothyroidism)
Too little thyroid hormone leads to gaining weight, feeling tired. . .
High antibodies means thyroid is being attacked-can be autoimmune problem

(handwritten annotation at bottom)
*****will need medicine to replace T4 I'm not making!

pituitary is sending lots of TSH (Thyroid Stimulating Hormone is too high) to it, telling the thyroid to make more thyroid hormone. This can happen when the thyroid stops working because antibodies are attacking it. Sally's antibody levels are really high. Having high levels of antibodies attacking the thyroid can be an autoimmune problem. Sally's own immune system is attacking her thyroid. This is a fairly common problem. Sally will need to take medicine to replace the thyroid hormone she is not making herself (probably for the rest of her life). Her doctor should be able to explain all of this to Sally so she can understand what she needs to do. Sally can take notes at her doctor's office (like those added to her test results) or add them at a later time if she needs to look up any more information. Sally could find out much more about her thyroid problem using some of the resources listed in Chapter 4.

CASE STUDY

Urine Test

The second test results are for Dawn Jones. Dawn went to her doctor because she was having pain after urinating (peeing). Her doctor sent her to have a urine test done to check and see if she had a urinary tract infection. Dawn's test results are shown on the next two pages. The first page shows her original results as obtained from her doctor, while the second page has notes added to explain her results.

Dawn's urine test results have three main test areas that are listed under test name in the upper left hand corner. The three main types of tests run were:

❖ Urinalysis (testing for many different items in urine).

❖ Urine culture (try to see if anything in the urine like bacteria will grow).

❖ Susceptibility (if bacteria do grow, then different drugs are tested to see which ones will kill the bacteria).

ACCURATE LABORATORY
123 LAB STREET
ANYTOWN, USA 12345
(123) 456-7899

DR. LAB BOSS, M.D.

PATIENT NAME: DAWN JONES

PATIENT AGE: 34

PATIENT SEX: F

DR. I CAN HELP
333 COMFORT LANE
HOMETOWN, MI 12345

PATIENT I.D. NO.   123456789

TIME OF REPORT   3:00PM

DATE OF REPORT   8/14/03

DATE OF SPECIMEN   8/11/03

DATE RECEIVED   8/11/03

TIME COLLECTED   10:00AM

TEST NAME	REFERENCE RANGE	RESULT	ABNORMAL	UNITS
URINALYSIS, URINE CULTURE, SUSCEPTIBILITY				
URINALYSIS:				
COLOR		YELLOW		
APPEARANCE		CLEAR		
SPECIFIC GRAVITY	1.005-1.030	1.010		
PH	5.0-7.5	6		
PROTEIN	NEG/TRACE	NEG		
GLUCOSE	NEG	NEG		
KETONES	NEG	NEG		
BILIRUBIN	NEG	NEG		
BLOOD	NEG	2		
RBC	0-3		5-10	/HPF
WBC	0-5	NONE		/HPF
EPITHELIAL CELLS	0-5	FEW		
2+ BACTERIA:				
LEUKOCYTE ESTERASE			TRACE	
NITRITE	NEG	NEG		
URINE CULTURE, ROUTINE:				
FINAL RESULT:				

COLONY COUNT: >=100,000 CFU/ML
PSEUDOMONAS AERUGINOSA
MULTIPLE ORGANISMS PRESENT—SUSCEPTIBILITY PERFORMED ON PREDOMINANT
ORGANISM(S) ONLY

SUSCEPTIBILITY:

SUSCEPTIBILITY	1	2	3	4	SUSCEPTIBILITY	1	2	3	4
AMPICILLIN	R	—	—	—	CARBENICILLIN	S	—	—	—
CEFTRIAXONE	S	—	—	—	CEPHALOTHIN	R	—	—	—
CIPROFLOXACIN	S	—	—	—	GENTAMICIN	S	—	—	—
NALADIXIC ACID	R	—	—	—	NITROFURANTOIN	R	—	—	—
NORFLOXACIN	S	—	—	—	TETRACYCLINE	I	—	—	—
TOBRAMYCIN	S	—	—	—	TREMETH/SULFA	R	—	—	—

ACCURATE LABORATORY
123 LAB STREET
ANYTOWN, USA 12345
(123) 456-7899

DR. LAB BOSS, M.D.

PATIENT NAME:	DAWN JONES	PATIENT I.D. NO.	123456789
PATIENT AGE:	34	TIME OF REPORT	3:00PM
PATIENT SEX:	F	DATE OF REPORT	8/14/03
		DATE OF SPECIMEN	8/11/03
DR. I CAN HELP		DATE RECEIVED	8/11/03
333 COMFORT LANE		TIME COLLECTED	10:00AM
HOMETOWN, MI 12345			

TEST NAME	REFERENCE RANGE	RESULT	ABNORMAL	UNITS
URINALYSIS, URINE CULTURE, SUSCEPTIBILITY				
URINALYSIS:				
COLOR		YELLOW		
APPEARANCE		CLEAR		
SPECIFIC GRAVITY	1.005-1.030	1.010		
PH	5.0-7.5	6		
PROTEIN	NEG/TRACE	NEG		
GLUCOSE	NEG	NEG		
KETONES	NEG	NEG		
BILIRUBIN	NEG	NEG		
BLOOD	NEG	2		
RBC	0-3		5-10	/HPF
WBC	0-5	NONE		/HPF
EPITHELIAL CELLS	0-5	FEW		
2+ BACTERIA:				
LEUKOCYTE ESTERASE			TRACE	
NITRITE	NEG	NEG		

Results are out of normal ranges.

URINE CULTURE, ROUTINE:
FINAL RESULT:

COLONY COUNT: >=100,000 CFU/ML
PSEUDOMONAS AERUGINOSA
MULTIPLE ORGANISMS PRESENT—SUSCEPTIBILITY PERFORMED ON PREDOMINANT ORGANISM(S) ONLY

Type and amount of bacteria causing infection

SUSCEPTIBILITY:

SUSCEPTIBILITY	1	2	3	4	SUSCEPTIBILITY	1	2	3	4
AMPICILLIN	R	—	—	—	CARBENICILLIN	S	—	—	—
CEFTRIAXONE	S	—	—	—	CEPHALOTHIN	R	—	—	—
CIPROFLOXACIN	S	—	—	—	GENTAMICIN	S	—	—	—
NALADIXIC ACID	R	—	—	—	NITROFURANTOIN	R	—	—	—
NORFLOXACIN	S	—	—	—	TETRACYCLINE	I	—	—	—
TOBRAMYCIN	S	—	—	—	TREMETH/SULFA	R	—	—	—

Bacteria are resistant (still live) or are susceptible (are killed) by these drugs.

While there is a great deal of information on Dawn's test reports, the important thing to concentrate on are any results that are abnormal or out of the normal range. Dawn's doctor told her she had a urinary tract infection (bladder infection) and she would need to take antibiotic medicine for ten days. The abnormal results under urinalysis for extra RBC (red blood cells) and the trace presence of leukocyte esterase let Dawn's doctor know an infection was present. The urine culture results told Dr. I Can Help that Dawn's infection was due to more than one bacterium, but the main bacteria was *pseudomonas aeruginosa*. This bacteria was present in high numbers with over 100,000 colonies/milliliter of urine. Since a main bacterium was found, the lab went on to test for susceptibility.

Susceptibility testing is done to find a medication that will kill the specific bacteria and clear up Dawn's infection. An "R" under this section means that these drugs will not work to kill the bacteria (bacteria is resistant to the drug). An "S" under this section means that these drugs will kill the bacteria (bacteria is susceptible to the drug). Incidentally, the "I" under this section for Tetracycline means that test results could not be shown to be either resistant or susceptible (in this case the test result is indeterminate or cannot be determined). A drug that is shown to be indeterminate would not be considered as a treatment drug. So, Dawn's doctor can pick one of the drugs listed on her lab report with an "S" to prescribe for her to clear up her infection.

It is not uncommon for women to have occasional urinary infections, but if Dawn continues to have problems, or simply wants to find out more information on how to prevent them, she could ask her doctor for written information or she could use the resources found in Chapter 4.

CASE STUDY

MRI Test

The third test results are for Jason Memory. Jason went to his doctor because he was having trouble remembering things that used to be easy to remember. His doctor sent him to have an MRI of the brain. Jason's test results are shown on the next two pages. The first page shows his original results as obtained from his doctor, while the second page has notes added to explain his results.

Jason's test results are complicated to read and understand because of all the medical terms the average person cannot be expected to know. When you have test results like this you need to forget trying to understand every word and concentrate on what your doctor tells you. You should also make sure you get the following questions answered:

✤ What did the doctor suspect before he or she sent you for the test?

✤ What test was run?

✤ What were the important findings?

✤ What are the possible explanations or diagnoses?

✤ What recommendations were given?

These questions can be answered by looking at the test results with notes added. Near the top of the page is an area called "CLINICAL DIAGNOSIS." The words "50 RO MULTIPLE SCLEROSIS" are typed in. This means that Jason's doctor sent him for the test to rule out (RO) multiple sclerosis. His doctor wanted the test done to make sure Jason didn't have multiple sclerosis. The name of the test run is just below this area where it reads "1 MRI BRAIN INCL STEM WITHOUT CONTRAST". This indicates that one MRI test

WECAREFORU HOSPITAL
123 HOSPITAL AVENUE
ANYTOWN, USA 12345
(123) 456-7899
RADIOLOGY REPORT
DR. BOSS, M.D.

PATIENT NAME: JASON MEMORY
PATIENT AGE: 32
PATIENT SEX: M

PATIENT I.D. NO. 123456789
TIME OF REPORT 7:39AM
DATE OF REPORT 3/13/96
DATE OF TEST 3/12/96

DR. I CAN HELP
333 COMFORT LANE
HOMETOWN, MI 12345

CLINICAL DIAGNOSIS
50 RO MULTIPLE SCLEROSIS

1 MRI BRAIN INCL STEM WITHOUT CONTRAST: No prior studies are available for comparison purposes.

Multi-planar, multi-sequential images of the brain are obtained.

The ventricles, basal cisterns and sulci over the convexities appear within normal limits for the patient's age. Mild signal abnormality within the ethmoid and maxillary sinuses is most likely related to inflammatory or post-inflammatory changes.

Mild inflammatory changes are also likely apparent in the sphenoid sinus. The cranioverte-bral junction and relationships appear intact. There are multiple foci of scattered abnormally increased signal intensity within the deep subcortical and periventricular white matter bilaterally. These create no mass effect and demonstrate no substantial surrounding edema and are of indeterminate etiology. Diagnostic considerations would include demyelinating processes possible secondary to multiple sclerosis or ischemia. These can also be seen in patient's with migraine headaches. Infectious or inflammatory etiologies could also not be excluded. Neoplasm would be much less likely. Clinical correlation is recommended.

IMPRESSION:
1. Scattered foci of abnormally increased signal intensity within the periventricular white matter. See above discussion. Diagnostic considerations would include multiple sclerosis as well as several other etiologies as described above and clinical correlation is recommended.
2. Inflammatory changes or post-inflammatory changes in the paranasal sinuses.

I. C. Ray, M.D.

ICR/mb

WECAREFORU HOSPITAL
123 HOSPITAL AVENUE
ANYTOWN, USA 12345
(123) 456-7899
RADIOLOGY REPORT
DR. BOSS, M.D.

PATIENT NAME: JASON MEMORY
PATIENT AGE: 32
PATIENT SEX: M

Rule out multiple sclerosis

PATIENT I.D. NO. 123456789
TIME OF REPORT 7:39AM
DATE OF REPORT 3/13/96
DATE OF TEST 3/12/96

DR. I CAN HELP
333 COMFORT LANE
HOMETOWN, MI 12345

CLINICAL DIAGNOSIS 50 RO MULTIPLE SCLEROSIS

Test run MRI of brain including brainstem

1 MRI BRAIN INCL STEM WITHOUT CONTRAST: No prior studies are available for comparison purposes.

Multi-planar, multi-sequential images of the brain are obtained.

The ventricles, basal cisterns and sulci over the convexities appear within normal limits for the patient's age. Mild signal abnormality within the ethmoid and maxillary sinuses is most likely related to inflammatory or post-inflammatory changes.

Mild inflammatory changes are also likely apparent in the sphenoid sinus. The craniovertebral junction and relationships appear intact. There are multiple foci of scattered abnormally increased signal intensity within the deep subcortical and periventricular white matter bilaterally. These create no mass effect and demonstrate no substantial surrounding edema and are of indeterminate etiology. Diagnostic considerations would include demyelinating processes possible secondary to multiple sclerosis or ischemia. These can also be seen in patient's with migraine headaches. Infectious or inflammatory etiologies could also not be excluded. Neoplasm would be much less likely. Clinical correlation is recommended.

Important to understand!!

IMPRESSION:

1. Scattered foci of abnormally increased signal intensity within the periventricular white matter. See above discussion. Diagnostic considerations would include multiple sclerosis as well as several other etiologies as described above and clinical correlation is recommended.
2. Inflammatory changes or post-inflammatory changes in the paranasal sinuses.

I. C. Ray, M.D.

ICR/mb

Diagnoses??
- multiple sclerosis
- ischemia
- migraines
- infection
- inflammation
- neoplasm

of the brain including the brainstem was done without contrast material (special dye).

The important findings can be found under the "IMPRESSION" area. The most important finding was "Scattered foci of abnormally increased signal intensity within the periventricular white matter." While this is the technical description (sometimes called UBOs for unidentified bright objects), the reality is that Jason had many more "spots" on the brain scan that weren't normally found on a man of his age. (The second finding under impression is less important and may mean Jason had a recent sinus infection.)

Possible diagnoses for the finding of the "spots" can be found underlined in the paragraph just above "IMPRESSION". Possible diagnoses are always important to find as well as what recommendations are made. Possible diagnoses include multiple sclerosis, ischemia (lack of blood flow), migraine headaches, infection, inflammation, or neoplasm (tumor). It is also important to pick up on the fact that neoplasm was thought by the doctor reporting the results to be less likely to be the real diagnosis.

Finally, the recommendation given was "Clinical correlation is recommended." What this really means is that this test cannot decide which of the possible diagnoses the right diagnosis is. The results of extra "spots" can be found in all of the possible diagnoses, so it will take more clinical investigating (history and testing) to decide which diagnosis is the best fit for Jason.

Many times, a test result gives only one part of the answer and more testing is needed to find out the rest of the story.

Unfortunately for Jason, his doctor did not look at all the possible diagnoses. His doctor told him he had multiple sclerosis and then referred him to a neurologist who decided he had migraines. Jason was uncomfortable with such different ideas so he sought third and fourth opinions about his possible diagnoses. You can read more about what happened to Jason in Chapter 5 under "Seeking Second and Third Opinions."

The important thing to take away from Jason's story is that a doctor should not interpret more from a test result than is possible. Jason's test result did not find one diagnosis, rather six different possible diagnoses were given. All of the different diagnoses should have been evaluated further before a final diagnosis was given (especially when the possible diagnoses were as serious as Jason's). Always ask the doctor directly what all the possible diagnoses are and compare them to what is written on the actual test results This is another reason why it is so important to get copies of your test results.

CASE STUDY

Biopsy

The fourth and final test results are for a biopsy. Joanne went to her doctor because she had a cough that was getting worse. Joanne was a cigarette smoker. The chest x-ray taken at this first appointment showed a "mass in the right lung." Joanne's doctor sent her the next day to see a pulmonologist (lung specialist) to see what the mass shown on the x-ray was. The pulmonologist recommended that a biopsy be done to see exactly what the mass indicated. Joanne's test results are shown on the next two pages. The first page shows her original results as obtained from her doctor, while the second page has notes added to explain her lung biopsy results.

Joanne's doctor did not have good news for her. Unfortunately, the biopsy confirmed that the mass seen earlier on her chest x-ray was lung cancer. This was a very serious diagnosis for Joanne. After hearing the word "cancer," she found it almost impossible to think about anything else that was said during this appointment.

WECAREFORU HOSPITAL
123 HOSPITAL AVENUE
ANYTOWN, USA 12345
(123) 456-7899
SURGICAL PATHOLOGY REPORT
DR. BOSS, M.D.

PATIENT NAME: JOANNE N. TIME	PATIENT I.D. NO.　3737373737
PATIENT AGE:　63	TIME OF REPORT　1:00P.M.
PATIENT SEX:　F	DATE OF REPORT　8/21/02
	DATE OF TEST　8/21/02

DR. I CAN HELP
333 COMFORT LANE
HOMETOWN, MI 12345

Diagnosis/History
Lung Cancer

Procedure
Flexible bronchoscopy

Specimen(s) Received
Bronchial biopsy, rt main stem

Final Pathologic Diagnosis
Transbronchial biopsy of right main stem bronchus:

Moderate to poorly differentiated squamous cell carcinoma.

A. Lab Doctor, M.D.

Gross Description

The specimen is labeled bronchial biopsy right main stem and consists of multiple fragments of soft pale white tissue aggregating to 9.0 x 3.0 x 2.0 mm. All submitted in one cassette.

A. Lab Doctor, M.D.

Microscopic Description

The sections demonstrate multiple fragments of malignant epithelium as well as portions of the apparent mucosa showing squamous metaplasia of the bronchial mucosa. The malignant fragments are comprised of moderately to markedly pleomorphic epidermoid cells showing enlarged, hyperchromatic nuclei and an increase in the nuclear to cytoplasmic ratio. Some of the cells appear to keratinize and mitotic figures are frequent. The tumor invades into the smooth muscle beneath the mucosa.

END OF REPORT

WECAREFORU HOSPITAL
123 HOSPITAL AVENUE
ANYTOWN, USA 12345
(123) 456-7899
SURGICAL PATHOLOGY REPORT
DR. BOSS, M.D.

PATIENT NAME: JOANNE N. TIME   PATIENT I.D. NO.   3737373737
PATIENT AGE: 63   TIME OF REPORT   1:00P.M.
PATIENT SEX: F   DATE OF REPORT   8/21/02
                                         DATE OF TEST   8/21/02

DR. I CAN HELP   (**Suspected diagnosis**)
333 COMFORT LANE
HOMETOWN, MI 12345

Diagnosis/History
Lung Cancer

(**Using a tube to see into the lungs (and to take a sample)**)

Procedure
Flexible bronchoscopy

(**Final diagnosis of squamous cell lung cancer.**)

Specimen(s) Received
Bronchial biopsy, rt main stem

Final Pathologic Diagnosis
Transbronchial biopsy of right main stem bronchus:
   Moderate to poorly differentiated squamous cell carcinoma.

                              A. Lab Doctor, M.D.

Gross Description

(**Location and size of sample taken.**)

The specimen is labeled bronchial biopsy right main stem and consists of multiple fragments of soft pale white tissue aggregating to 9.0 x 3.0 x 2.0 mm. All submitted in one cassette.

                              A. Lab Doctor, M.D.

Microscopic Description

The sections demonstrate multiple fragments of <u>malignant epithelium</u> as well as portions of the apparent mucosa showing squamous metaplasia of the bronchial mucosa. The malignant fragments are comprised of moderately to markedly <u>pleomorphic epidermoid cells</u> showing enlarged, <u>hyperchromatic nuclei</u> and an <u>increase in the nuclear to cytoplasmic ratio</u>. Some of the cells appear to keratinize and <u>mitotic figures</u> are frequent. The <u>tumor invades</u> into the smooth muscle beneath the mucosa.

END OF REPORT   (**Microscopic findings of cancer cells**)

Luckily for Joanne, two other family members had come with her to her appointment. They were able to listen closely to the rest of the information presented and remember what Joanne could not remember hearing.

Oftentimes, after hearing a serious diagnosis like "cancer," a patient will be unable to concentrate on anything else that is said during the appointment. Their focus stays on the word "cancer" and they often do not remember much about the rest of the appointment. This is why it's important to have a patient advocate present for any consultation appointments following serious procedures or biopsies. Patient advocates can help remember the rest of what was discussed and can help you keep the "bigger picture" in mind.

In addition, whenever cancer is found, it's really important to get a copy of the actual pathology report because it can tell you a lot more about the type of cancer present. Different types of cancer grow at different rates, respond to different treatments, and have different possible outcomes. Knowing as much as you can about the type of cancer present is important in helping to decide treatment and the best outcome.

In Joanne's case, because of the diagnosis of cancer, it's especially crucial to use her test results and the doctor's comments to answer the questions previously discussed for any test result:

❖ What did the doctor suspect before he or she sent you for the test?

❖ What test was run?

❖ What were the important findings?

❖ What are the possible explanations or diagnoses?

❖ What recommendations were given?

These questions can be answered by looking at Joanne's test results with notes added. Near the top of the page is an area called "Diagnosis/History" with the words "Lung Cancer" found directly below them. This shows that Joanne's doctor suspected she had lung cancer before the biopsy was performed. Her doctor suspected lung cancer because of the mass found on her chest x-ray and her history of cigarette smoking. Just below the words "Lung Cancer" the word "Procedure" appears. This area of the report tells you what test was run. Joanne had a flexible bronchoscopy done. During this test a flexible tube was inserted into the airway branches leading to Joanne's lungs. This test is done at a hospital under anesthesia. The bronchoscope (the tool used) lets the doctor see inside the airways and also allows the doctor the ability to take a sample biopsy of any suspicious areas.

The important finding in Joanne's test was the sampling of suspicious areas that were biopsied in the main stem (branch) of her right lung. This information is found on her results under "Gross Description." Incidentally, the word "Gross" here means looking at the sample(s) with the naked eye, not through any magnification. It does not mean anything distasteful. The samples all taken together measured 9.0 x 3.0 x 2.0 mm. The "Microscopic Description" can be found after the "Gross Description" on Joanne's results. The details of the microscopic description are the important findings because looking at the sample under the microscope lets the pathologist (lab doctor) know what type of cells are present and what condition they are in. This information is then used to decide upon a diagnosis. Many of the key terms are underlined in this section of Joanne's report to point out terms often used to describe cancer cells. These underlined terms describing cancer cells include:

✤ Malignant epithelium.

✤ Pleomorphic edpidermoid cells.

✤ Hyperchromatic nuclei.

✤ Increase in the nuclear to cytoplasmic ratio.

✤ Mitotic figures.

✤ Tumor invades.

While most of these terms are very technical, it's important to at least realize that the terms *malignant* and *tumor invades* refer to cancer cells. If you wanted to understand the rest of these terms, you could ask your doctor or look up the terms in a medical dictionary. Cancer is never a good diagnosis and "tumor invades" is even a worse sign because it means that the cancer cells are starting to invade deeper areas.

The pathologist used all of these findings and the type of cells looked at (epithelial — lining the airways) to come up with a "Final Pathologic Diagnosis" of "squamous cell carcinoma" of the right main stem brochus. In simpler terms this means squamous cell carcinoma of Joanne's right lung. This is a serious diagnosis, but much more information needs to be learned before any treatment can be recommended or any outcome can be predicted.

Finding cancer is one thing, but important questions need to be answered as quickly as possible. Specifically:

❖ Is the type of cancer slow or fast growing?

❖ How many areas of cancer are there?

❖ Is there any cancer in the lymph nodes?

❖ Has the cancer spread to any other areas?

Much more testing is needed to answer these types of questions. Most often a patient will be referred to an oncologist (cancer doctor) to help sort through these questions and determine treatment options. For these reasons, Joanne's report does not answer the last question: "What recommendations are given?" Recommendations cannot always be given from simply a biopsy result until much more information is learned.

What will happen to a patient with cancer depends on many factors, and being diagnosed with cancer does not always mean a death sentence. While it is difficult to do, the person diagnosed with cancer (and his or her family members and friends) need to find out all of the information possible before jumping to any conclusions. Today many types of cancer can be beaten. Even when cancer cannot be cured, there are many treatments that can extend life and/or improve the quality of life.

In Joanne's case, her biopsy results could only answer the first question listed above. Squamous cell carcinoma of the lung tends to be one of the more slowly growing types of lung cancer. This is an important fact because the speed with which cancer grows, together with when the cancer is first discovered, oftentimes makes all the difference in what will ultimately happen to a patient.

There is much more to Joanne's story than just her test results. Joanne was diagnosed with a life-threatening diagnosis of lung cancer, but the rest of her story may surprise you. You can read more about what happened to Joanne in Chapter 5 under "Seeking Second and

Third Opinions." The important thing to take away from Joanne's results is that she had a very serious diagnosis (lung cancer) given to her, but much more testing and information was needed before any treatment options or any outcomes could be predicted. Biopsies can help give a specific diagnosis, but they are often only one part of the big picture.

This section has shown you four different types of test results (blood, urine, MRI, and biopsy). While these tests varied greatly in the level of seriousness, they all demonstrated important points. Hopefully learning how to add notes to the test results helped you to simplify the information and to concentrate on the important areas. You can understand your test results, too, if you just look at the reports one section at a time and concentrate your efforts on the abnormal results and the important findings and diagnoses. Don't forget to ask your doctor any questions you may have. It's okay to be proactive in your own treatment. After all, this is part of being a SMART patient. Good Luck!

Prescription Drugs (Rx)

Millions and millions of people take prescription drugs everyday in the United States. This means that millions and millions of prescriptions are filled each day and the numbers continue to increase. In fact, a recent *U.S. News & World Report* article states that "between 1995 and 2003, the number of prescriptions sold each year in the United States rocketed up from 2.1 billion to 3.2 billion" (Querna, 2005). Although pharmacies try to fill these prescriptions carefully, errors occur. Sometimes the errors are caught before a drug is taken and sometimes they aren't. Some of the errors cause mild problems, and some can kill. Over 7000 people died in 1993 from medication errors: accidental poisoning by drugs, medicaments and biologicals that resulted from acknowledged errors by patients or medical personnel (Institute of Medicine, 2000; Philips, et al., 1998). If you do not want to suffer because you ended up with a different drug than what your doctor intended, or if it was the wrong drug prescribed for you in the first place, then you need to look out for yourself! Looking out for yourself with prescription drugs starts right at your doctor's office.

Before your doctor gives you a prescription for any medication, be sure he or she knows the following:

✤ Your complete medical history.

✤ Age (some medications aren't given to young children and some medication amounts need to be adjusted for children and the elderly).

✤ Weight (can affect how much medication is given especially in infants and young children).

✤ Any allergies you have (especially to medications and what happened when you were given these medications in the past).

✤ If you are pregnant or breastfeeding.

✤ Bad non-allergic reactions (side effects) you've had to past medications.

✤ All other medications you are taking (both prescription and what you buy over the counter).

✤ Any vitamins or supplements (like herbs) you are taking.

✤ Immunization record (i.e., flu vaccine, tetanus vaccine, etc.).

All of this information is vitally important when deciding the best drug for your particular problem and to make sure the new drug will not cause a bad reaction with other drugs or supplements you are taking. Review this information with your doctor each time you get a new prescription. You may be taking new medicines since the last time you saw your doctor. You should also make sure the pharmacy where you have your prescriptions filled knows this information. Pharmacies use computer programs to help make sure you do not take medicines that could react badly with other drugs or supplements you may be taking.

It may be difficult for you to remember what you are currently taking and what you are allergic to, so it's a good idea to keep a list with you. If you keep a current list of your medications and your allergies, you can then give your doctor the most current information. This list should include information like:

> *Don't assume your doctor knows what you are allergic to or what medications/supplements/ vitamins you are currently taking because it's in the chart. The reality is that doctors do not read your entire chart each time they see you. They might not realize what medications you are taking or what you are allergic to unless you refresh their memory. This is very important to do.*

- ❖ Specific names of medicines you take (including strength and form).

- ❖ How often you take the medicines.

- ❖ When you first started taking the medicines (hours/days/weeks/ months or years ago).

- ❖ Any vitamins, over-the-counter medicines, herbs, or supplements you take.

- ❖ Any allergies you have (especially drug allergies).

✤ Bad non-allergic reactions to past medications (side effects).

✤ Name and phone number of your pharmacy.

This list doesn't need to be fancy, but it does need to be accurate. Remember to look out for yourself! The *My Medications* form can be used to write down all the medications, vitamins, and supplements you currently take. An example of a completed *My Medications* form can be found on the next page. Be sure to update this form as you start or stop new medications. (For photocopying purposes, a blank *My Medications* form can be found in Appendix 1.)

Two good reasons why you should keep a list of prescription drugs you are taking:

1. *You need to understand about the drug you will be taking, and*

2. *You can use the information to help ensure you get the right prescription from your pharmacist.*

My Medications

Your Name: <u>IMA Smart Patient</u>

Doctor's Name / Phone #: <u>I Can Help, M.D. / 313-321-3000</u>

Pharmacy's Name / Phone #: <u>Corner Drugstore / 313-333-3333</u>

Today's Date: <u>April 14, 2003</u>

1. Current medication(s) (name, strength, form, how often taken, when started):

Name	Strength	Form	How often	When started
Nexium®	40mg	capsule	one/day before breakfast	Nov. 2003
Centrum®	multi-vitamin	tablet	one/day with lunch	years ago
Tums®	XS	tablet	2 tablets/ day	since thyroid surgery
Levoxyl®	125 mcg	tablet	one/day at bedtime	since thyroid surgery

2. Allergy(allergies) and reaction(s)(what happened, when): _____

<u>Penicillin — body rash as baby</u>

<u>Clindamycin — chest rash as adult</u>

<u>Latex allergy since 1996 — rashes, watery eyes, runny</u>

<u>nose, tickle in throat</u>

3. Bad non-allergic reaction(s) to a medication(s) (medication & what happened):

<u>Vicodin® — dizzy and sick to stomach</u>

<u>Erythromycin — diarrhea</u>

When you are given a *new* prescription drug from your doctor, make sure you write down certain drug information. This information should include:

✢ The name of the drug (brand name and generic).

✢ The strength or dosage.

✢ The form of the drug (tablet, capsule, cream, ointment, solution, suspension, etc.).

✢ How many/much medication is being given (# pills, amt. liquid, etc.).

✢ Instructions for taking the medication (once per day, twice per day with meals, etc.).

✢ Is a generic substitute drug okay?

✢ Are there any refills available?

✢ How long will I need to be on this drug?

✢ Can I just call if I need refills or will I need to see the doctor again?

The *My New Rx Medication* form on pages 112 and 113 will help you to get this drug information from your doctor quickly. Double-check that you have the correct spelling of the drug you are to be given and know what type of drug it is. If you may receive the generic form of the drug, be sure to know both the brand name and the generic name. You should know what form the drug is in. Is it a tablet, a capsule, a cream, or a liquid? If it's a liquid, is it a solution or a suspension? The same drug created as a solution or a suspension can have different effects on a patient. It is important that you know which form of the medication your doctor wants you to have so you get the same form from the pharmacist. If your doctor prescribes a suspension, then make sure you get a suspension. This can help prevent you from getting the wrong drug from the pharmacist.

Your doctor and his staff should be willing to help you fill out the form *My New Rx Medication*. If not, then you need to ask yourself if you are in the right office. After all, physicians are supposed to answer your questions and help you understand your care, right? The form is easy to read and should not take longer than a few minutes to complete. An example of a completed *My New Rx Medication* form can be found on the next page. (For photocopying purposes, a blank *My New Rx Medication* form can be found in Appendix 1.)

My New Rx Medication *(page 1)*

Your Name: __IMA Smart Patient__

Doctor's Name: __I Can Help, M.D.__

Doctor's Phone #: __313-321-3000__

Today's Date: __April 20, 2004__

1. Name, strength and form of new medication (be specific): _____

__Levoxyl® 125 mcg (thyroid medication)__

_____

2. Amount of medication given per prescription (oz., # of pills, etc.): _____

__30 tablets__

_____

3. Instructions for taking the medication:

(Take by mouth)   Apply to problem area

Do not chew   Avoid exposure to sunlight

Be careful about rising too fast after lying down

Take with food   (Take on an empty stomach)

__(1 hour before or 2-3 hours after a meal)__

Avoid alcohol   Store: In the refrigerator   At room temperature

Avoid __calcium__ foods or __antacids, iron, vitamin__ medicines within

__4__ hours of taking this medication.

Take in the morning   Take at bedtime

(Once/day)   Twice/day   Three times/day   Four times/day

__Take same time of day, every day__

My New Rx Medication *(page 2)*

4. Is a generic version of the medicine all right to use?

(No)   Yes

5. How long will I need to be on this medicine? _____

Will need thyroid replacement drugs for the rest of my
life (even though exact dosage may change).
_____

6. Are there refills available?

No   (Yes) __5__ times

Can I call your office if I need refills or will I need another appointment

with you? _____

_____

_____

_____

_____

7. Do I need to have my blood checked while on this medicine?

If yes, how often? _Yes, every 4-6 weeks for first few_
months, then every 6 months.
_____

_____

_____

_____

_____

_____

Sometimes drug names are very similar and if the pharmacist cannot read the prescription because of poor handwriting or miscommunication over the phone (remember the telephone game as a child?), sometimes the wrong drug is given. In fact, there are hundreds and hundreds of drug names that can be confused with each other. Even though the drug names may look alike or sound alike, everything else about each of these drugs can be very different. These drugs can be totally different with respect to chemical make-ups, effects on a patient, and reasons for prescribing them in the first place. These differences can cause serious problems for a patient and in severe cases even cause death. Examples of some drug names that can be easily confused are:

There are many drugs that can look alike (with poor handwriting) or sound alike (on the phone). In order to make sure you are getting the right drug for you, use the form **"My New Rx Medication"**!

Ceftin® vs. Cefzil®

Celebrex® vs. Celexa®

Chlorpromazine vs. Chlorpropamide

Dopamine vs. Dobutamine

Hydrocodone vs. Hydrocortisone

Paxil® vs. Taxol®

Prednisone vs. Prednisolone

Slobid® vs. Lobid®

Tobrex® vs. Tobradex®

Vistaril® vs. Restoril®

Xanax® vs. Zantac®

Zyrtec® vs. Zyprexa®

These are just a few of the hundreds of current confusing drug names. A much more comprehensive listing of look-alike, sound-alike drug names can be found under "Patient Safety" at www.usp.org. This is the website for the United States Pharmacopeia, a collected body of information on the standards of strength, purity, and quality of drugs in the United States.

If you don't like to fill out forms and you would rather try to understand the prescription form your doctor gave you, go ahead. Just remember, it's often hard to read a doctor's handwriting and it takes more effort than filling out the previous form. If you choose to do this, though, here are some helpful hints. First understand that you *can* recognize the basic parts of a prescription. Below are the items you will find on a prescription form. The three items most important for figuring out what drug you are being asked to take have a box surrounding where they are located on the prescription form on the next page. All prescriptions list:

❖ Your name and address.

❖ Your age (if needed).

❖ Your weight (if needed, especially for infant or young child).

❖ The date.

❖ Your doctor's name and address.

❖ Your doctor's license number (state medical or dental license number).

✤ Your doctor's DEA number (needed for some types of drugs). A DEA number is required on a prescription when the drug prescribed is a controlled drug as listed by the Controlled Substances Act of 1970 (U.S.). Each doctor who prescribes controlled drugs will have their own DEA number.

✤ Rx (sign): next to this sign, the name and strength of the medication is written (see upper box surrounding this information on the next page).

✤ Disp. (Dispense): this line tells you how much of the medication is being given (see middle box surrounding this information on the next page).

✤ Sig. (Signatura): these lines give you instructions on how and when to take the medication (see lower box surrounding this information on the next page).

✤ D.A.W.: stands for dispense as written. When this is written on a prescription the specific drug requested must be given — no generic drugs can be substituted. If D.A.W. is not written and there is another drug equivalent to what was prescribed, then the pharmacist can dispense the generic drug instead of what was requested.

✤ Refills: tells you if you can refill this prescription again or not.

On the next page is a blank prescription form with boxes added to show you where you will find the three important items for figuring out what and how much of a medicine you are being given.

NAME OF YOUR DOCTOR'S OFFICE
YOUR DOCTOR, M.D.
YOUR DOCTOR'S PARTNER, M.D.
123 STREET
ANYTOWN, USA 12345

#(123) 456-7899   DEA# _____
                                                        LIC# _____

NAME _____ AGE _____

ADDRESS _____ DATE _____

Rx

> Name & Strength of Medicine

> Disp: Amount of Medicine Given

> Sig: Instructions on When & How to Take Medicine

Refill _____ times

_____
(signature)

Another brand of generically equivalent product, identical
in dosage, form and content of active ingredients, may
be dispensed unless box is initialed D.A.W.

Sometimes everything on a prescription is written out in long-hand, but many times abbreviations are used. Some of the common abbreviations used by doctors and pharmacists are listed in Table 2 (Hooley and Whitacre, 1984; *Mosby Medical Dictionary,* 2002; *Stedman's Medical Dictionary,* 1982; *Merriam-Webster's Collegiate Dictionary,* 2004).

Prescription Abbreviations

Table 2

ABBREVIATION	MEANING	LATIN
a.c.	before meals	ante cibum
aa or AA	of each	ana
ad	up to	ad
aq.	water	aqua
aur.	the ear, ears	auris, aures
b.i.d.	twice a day	bis in die
c.	with	cum
cib.	food, meal	cibus
f.	make	fac
ft.	let be made	fiat
gt. or gtt.	drop, drops	gutta, guttae
h.s.	at bedtime	hora somni
int. cib.	between meals	inter cibos
m.	mix	misce
non rep.	do not repeat	ne repetatur
O.D.	right eye	oculo dextro
O.S.	left eye	oculo sinistro
O.U.	in each eye	oculo utro
p.c.	after meals	post cibum
p.o.	take by mouth	per os

ABBREVIATION	MEANING	LATIN
p.r.n.	when needed	pro re nata
q. 2 h.	every two hours	quaque secunda hora
q. 3 h.	every three hours	quaque tertia hora
q. 4 h.	every four hours	quaque quarta hora
q.__°	every __ hour	quaque __ hora
q.d.	once a day	quaque die
q.h.	every hour	quaque hora
q.i.d.	four times a day	quarter in die
q.s.	a sufficient quantity	quantum sufficit
s.	without	sine
sig.	"let it be labeled"	signa or signatura
ss.	one half	semissem
stat	immediately	statim
T̄ or i	one	unus
t.i.d.	three times a day	ter in die
T̄T̄ or ii	two	duo
T̄T̄T̄ or iii	three	tres
ung.	ointment	unguentum
ut dict.	as directed	ut dictum

Prescription abbreviations not found on this list can be found by looking them up in medical dictionaries. Some medical dictionaries may even have an appendix listing many prescription abbreviations all in one place.

SAMPLE PRESCRIPTION

Below is a sample prescription. The sample shows how the prescription would be given to a patient.

NAME OF YOUR DOCTOR'S OFFICE
D. KNOWLEDGE, M.D.
YOUR DOCTOR'S PARTNER, M.D.
123 STREET
ANYTOWN, USA 12345

#(123) 456-7899

DEA# AK2345678

LIC# 891234

NAME *Joe Patient*   AGE *38*

ADDRESS *123 Everyday Lane*   DATE *8-11-03*

Hometown, MI 34567

Rx

Nasacort Nasal Spray

Disp: #1

Sig: ꚍ̄ spray each nostril q.d. prn

Refill *5* times

DKnowledge, MD
(signature)

Another brand of generically equivalent product, identical in dosage, form and content of active ingredients, may be dispensed unless box is initialed D.A.W.

The prescription form on the next page shows you what three main text lines to look at when trying to understand your prescription. Boxes surround the indicated lines of text.

Inside the upper box you will find the name and strength of the medication. Inside the middle box is how much medication is being given or dispensed. Inside the lower box are the instructions on how and when to take this medication. Once you have found these three lines of text on the prescription form, then you need to use the abbreviation list to understand any abbreviations you find. The prescription form on page 122 shows how to circle the abbreviations and add their meanings.

NAME OF YOUR DOCTOR'S OFFICE
D. KNOWLEDGE, M.D.
YOUR DOCTOR'S PARTNER, M.D.
123 STREET
ANYTOWN, USA 12345

#(123) 456-7899   DEA# AK2345678

LIC# 891234

NAME Joe Patient   AGE 38

ADDRESS 123 Everyday Lane   DATE 8-11-03

Hometown, MI 34567

Rx

Nasacort Nasal Spray

Disp: #1

Sig: Ť spray each nostril q.d. prn

Refill 5 times

DKnowledge, MD

(signature)

Another brand of generically equivalent product, identical
in dosage, form and content of active ingredients, may
be dispensed unless box is initialed D.A.W.

In this example, Dr. Knowledge has prescribed Nasacort® Nasal Spray for Joe Patient. Nasacort is used to treat allergies. Since it only comes in one dosage, there is no specific dosage next to the Rx sign. The dispense (Disp.) line shows that one bottle of spray is being prescribed at a time. The signature (Sig.) line gives the pharmacist the instructions for how Joe is to use the medication. Joe is supposed to use one (T̄) spray in each nostril every day (q.d.) when needed (prn). So Joe is to use the medication once per day when he is having problems with his allergies. Dr. Knowledge did not write D.A.W.

NAME OF YOUR DOCTOR'S OFFICE
YOUR DOCTOR, M.D.
YOUR DOCTOR'S PARTNER, M.D.
123 STREET
ANYTOWN, USA 12345

#(123) 456-7899   DEA# _____
                                       LIC# _____

NAME **Joe Patient**   AGE **38**

ADDRESS **123 Everyday Lane**   DATE **8-11-03**
              Hometown, MI 34567

Rx

     Nasacort Nasal Spray   "every day"

     Disp: #1 → "give one"

     Sig: T̄ spray each nostril q.d. prn.

          "one"   "when needed"

Refill **5** times

DKnowledge, MD
(signature)

Another brand of generically equivalent product, identical in dosage, form and content of active ingredients, may be dispensed unless box is initialed D.A.W.

on the form so Joe could be given a generic equivalent of this drug. However, since there is no generic equivalent for Nasacort®, Joe will actually get Nasacort® when he picks up his prescription. Joe can refill this prescription up to five times in one year. Usually, prescriptions must be filled within a year from the date they are written. After this time a new prescription is needed.

The next example is a sample prescription for Levoxyl®. The form below is how the prescription would be given to a patient, while the form on page 124 shows how to understand the important abbreviations.

NAME OF YOUR DOCTOR'S OFFICE
I CAN HELP, M.D.
SO CAN I HELP, M.D.
333 COMFORT LANE
HOMETOWN, MI 12345

#(123) 456-7899

DEA# AK3335555

LIC# 777888

NAME **Sally Tired**   AGE **30**

ADDRESS **456 Everyday Lane**   DATE **8-20-03**
Hometown, MI 45678

Rx

Levoxyl 125mcg

Disp: #30 tabs

Sig: †̄ tab q.d. on empty stomach

Refill **5** times

I Can Help, MD
(signature)

Another brand of generically equivalent product, identical in dosage, form and content of active ingredients, may be dispensed unless box is initialed D.A.W.

In this example, Dr. I Can Help has prescribed Levoxyl® for Sally Tired. Levoxyl® is a synthetic thyroid medication given to people who have hypothyroidism (low thyroid hormones due to disease, radiation, or surgery). Since Levoxyl® comes in many different dosages, there is a specific dosage of 125mcg written next to the Rx sign. The dispense (Disp.) line shows that 30 tablets are being prescribed

NAME OF YOUR DOCTOR'S OFFICE
I CAN HELP, M.D.
SO CAN I HELP, M.D.
333 COMFORT LANE
HOMETOWN, MI 12345

#(123) 456-7899

DEA# AK3335555

LIC# 777888

NAME **Sally Tired**   AGE **30**

ADDRESS **456 Everyday Lane**   DATE **8-20-03**
Hometown, MI 45678

Rx

Levoxyl 125mcg

Disp: (#30 tabs) → "give thirty tablets"

Sig: (T) tab (q.d.) on empty stomach

"one"

"tablet"

"every day"

Refill **5**

I Can Help, MD

(signature)

Another brand of generically equivalent product, identical in dosage, form and content of active ingredients, may be dispensed unless box is initialed D.A.W.

at a time. The signature (Sig.) line gives the pharmacist the instructions for how Sally is to use the medication. Sally is supposed to take one (T̄) tablet (tab) everyday (q.d.) on an empty stomach. (More of the Levoxyl® is absorbed by the body on an empty stomach.) Dr. I Can Help did not write D.A.W. on the form so Sally could be given a generic equivalent of this drug. Levoxyl® is actually a brand name of levothyroxine sodium made by Jones Pharma Incorporated. There are several different companies that make levothyroxine sodium tablets. However, it is better if patients taking thyroid hormone supplements always take the drug made by the same company. Sally can refill this prescription up to five times in one year.

A third and final prescription example for Motrin® is shown on pages 126 and 127. The prescription is first shown as the patient would receive it and then again with the abbreviations explained. In this example, Dr. I Can Help has prescribed Motrin® for patient Hada Surgery. Motrin® is a pain medication often given to people after surgery. Since Motrin® comes in many different dosages, there is a specific dosage of 600 mg tablet written next to the Rx sign. The dispense (Disp.) line shows that 50 tablets are being prescribed at a time. The signature (Sig.) line gives the pharmacist the instructions for how Hada is to use the medication. Hada is supposed to take one (T̄) tablet by mouth (p.o.) every 6 hours (q.6h.) when needed (p.r.n.) for pain. Dr. I Can Help did not write D.A.W. on the form so Sally could be given a generic equivalent of this drug. Motrin® is actually a brand name of ibuprofen 600 mg tablet. There are several different companies that make ibuprofen tablets. Hada can refill this prescription one time in one year.

```
┌─────────────────────────────────────────────────────────────┐
│                 NAME OF YOUR DOCTOR'S OFFICE                  │
│                      I CAN HELP, M.D.                         │
│                     SO CAN I HELP, M.D.                       │
│                      333 COMFORT LANE                         │
│                     HOMETOWN, MI  12345                       │
│   #(123) 456-7899              DEA# AK3335555                 │
│                               LIC#  777888                    │
│  ═══════════════════════════════════════════════════════════ │
│                                                               │
│   NAME  Hada Surgery                       AGE 56             │
│                                                               │
│   ADDRESS  234 Sunny Lane          DATE  4-12-04              │
│            Hometown, MI  56789                                │
│   Rx                                                          │
│                                                               │
│       Motrin 600 mg tablet                                    │
│                                                               │
│       Disp: #50                                               │
│                                                               │
│       Sig: T̄ tablet p.o. q.6h. p.r.n. pain                   │
│                                                               │
│                                                               │
│   Refill  1   times                                           │
│                                                               │
│                    I Can Help, MD                             │
│            ──────────────────────────────                     │
│                      (signature)                              │
│   Another brand of generically equivalent product, identical  │
│   in dosage, form and content of active ingredients, may     │
│   be dispensed unless box is initialed D.A.W.    ┌────────┐   │
│                                                  └────────┘   │
└─────────────────────────────────────────────────────────────┘
```

You are certainly encouraged to understand as best you can the actual prescriptions from your doctor's office. However, if you are going to practice interpreting the abbreviations, do not write on the actual prescription. Writing on the prescription, even if you are just trying to understand it, could be mistaken for altering a prescription (something you never should do). Either make a copy of the prescription and then make your notes on it or simply write all your

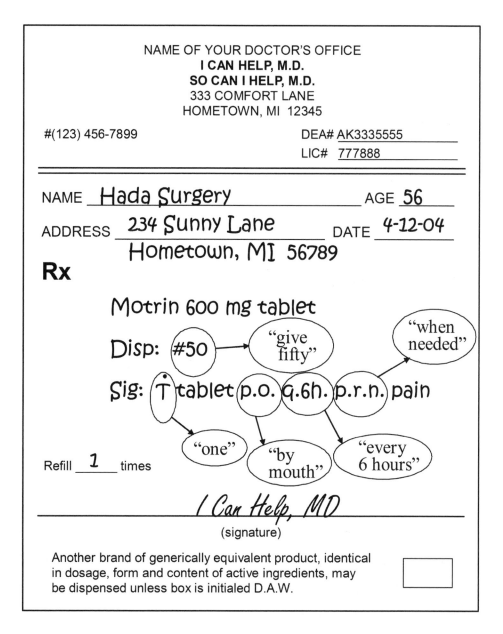

NAME OF YOUR DOCTOR'S OFFICE
I CAN HELP, M.D.
SO CAN I HELP, M.D.
333 COMFORT LANE
HOMETOWN, MI 12345

#(123) 456-7899

DEA# AK3335555

LIC# 777888

NAME Hada Surgery   AGE 56

ADDRESS 234 Sunny Lane   DATE 4-12-04
Hometown, MI 56789

Rx

Motrin 600 mg tablet

Disp: #50 → "give fifty"   "when needed"

Sig: T̈ tablet p.o. q.6h. p.r.n. pain

"one"   "by mouth"   "every 6 hours"

Refill 1 times

I Can Help, MD
(signature)

Another brand of generically equivalent product, identical
in dosage, form and content of active ingredients, may
be dispensed unless box is initialed D.A.W.

notes on another piece of paper. Even if you choose to interpret
your prescriptions, you still should use the *My New Rx Medication
Form* to make sure you know what your doctor wants you to take
before you leave your doctor's office. Making sure you understand
your doctor's instructions is more important than recognizing what
abbreviations are on the prescription.

Never try to adjust or modify a drug prescription you are given. Do not write on the actual prescription. Altering a drug prescription in any way (increasing the number of pills given, changing the refill number) is fraud. Altering drug prescriptions is illegal, dangerous, and may be punishable by fines and/or imprisonment.

Filling Your Prescription

Once you understand what medication your doctor wants you to take and how to take it, you will need to get this medication from your pharmacist. Pharmacists fill a lot of prescriptions each day and occasionally they make mistakes. Mistakes may happen when there is miscommunication between your doctor's office and the pharmacy, so it's always a good idea to check that you're getting the medication your doctor intended. How can you be sure of this? The following tips will help:

Tip #1

If possible, get your new prescriptions in writing to take to the pharmacy to be filled. While it is not as convenient for you, it does prevent phone errors between your doctor's office and your pharmacy. Sometimes the wrong medication or dosage is given to a patient because of miscommunication on the telephone. This happens more often than you might think. Do you remember playing the game "telephone" as a child? One child will whisper to another child who will repeat the same thing to another child and so on until the last child says out loud what he or she heard. Remember how the end story never matched the beginning one? It can happen with prescriptions called in over the phone, too.

Prescription miscommunication over the telephone can also be the result of a less experienced person calling in the prescription from the doctor's office. Doctors do not call in all the prescriptions they order. Oftentimes a nurse or even a receptionist will call in a prescription to a pharmacy. If the person making the call is not trained/experienced with a particular medication, sometimes the wrong information can be given to the pharmacy.

Prescription miscommunication happened to a thirty-something young woman with a urinary tract infection. Her doctor prescribed:

❖ 200 mg tablets of the antibiotic Floxin® to be taken every 12 hours for 10 days.

Instead of getting the correct drug from the pharmacy, she was given:

❖ 20 mg tablets of the muscle relaxant Flexeril® to be taken every 12 hours for 10 days.

By having the prescription filled over the phone the wrong drug was given. Luckily, the young woman was smart enough to look up the medication she was given in a PDR® (Physician's Desk Reference — a book containing information about prescription drugs). When she realized that she had been given a muscle relaxant instead of an antibiotic, she called her doctor. He had her write down exactly what he wanted her to take. After waiting for her doctor to phone in a new prescription (since it was after the doctor's office hours), she picked it up and compared it to exactly what her physician had told her she should be taking. In this case, both the doctor and the pharmacy blamed each other for the error. The young woman was smart enough to have discovered the error before she took any muscle relaxant, which would not have helped her urinary tract infection at all.

Tip #2

Try to have all your prescriptions filled at the same pharmacy. Pharmacies have computer programs that can check for drug interactions between different medicines being taken at the same time. This can be very important in preventing someone from taking drugs together that shouldn't be taken together. However, in order for this to work, the pharmacy needs to know all medications, vitamins, and supplements you are taking. Having your prescriptions filled at one pharmacy also allows medical providers access to all your medication information from one source. This can save valuable time and confusion. However, if you cannot have your prescriptions filled at the same pharmacy, then at least make sure each pharmacy knows all the drugs, vitamins, and supplements you are taking.

Tip #3

Find a pharmacy that uses a labeling system on their prescription, which identifies the medicine inside. While this may not be easy, it's a great tool in helping you obtain the medicine in the pill bottle that you are supposed to get. This labeling system prints out an extra label next to the usual prescription instructions and lets you know what your medicine should look like. This extra information may include the color, shape, and markings of the medicine. For example, a prescription written for propranolol 20mg tablets by Pliva would have extra information stating that the tablets are round, lt (light) blue, and marked with PLIVA 468. Comparing the information on the label to what is in the bottle is then easy to do. If the information doesn't match what is in the bottle, then you should immediately speak to the pharmacist. This is a wonderful system that unfortunately isn't available everywhere. You can call different pharmacies (retail chains, solely owned, outpatient hospital) to see if they use such a system.

Tip #4

If the medication comes in its original packaging, you can compare it to your notes on *My New Rx Medication* form. It should be fairly easy to make sure you have the right medication. If you are given a generic drug, you may have to compare the listed ingredients, not just the name.

Tip #5

If the medication does not come in the original packaging, but it is not generic, then you can look up the name of the drug in a pill book or a PDR® (Physicians Desk Reference). These books will help you find a description of the medication and/or sometimes a picture. In order to do this you need to make sure you are using the name of the company who made the drug. Different companies use different markings on their pills. You can check to make sure your pill matches in color, shape, size, and markings on each side.

Tip #6

If the medication does not come in the original packaging, but it is generic, then you can look up the name of the generic drug in a pill book or a PDR that contains generic drug information. These books are available at the library. If you have your prescriptions filled at a pharmacy that is part of a chain like RiteAid® or Walgreen®, you can call another pharmacy and ask them what the your medication should look like. You need to make sure the pharmacy you call is part of the same chain or they may not carry the drug made by the same company as the one you received. Again, you can check to see if your pill matches in color, shape, size, and markings on each side.

Tip #7

If you are simply refilling a prescription, be sure your new pills match the old pills you have been taking. If they do not match exactly, then you need find out why. You may have been given a different company's pills or you may have the wrong drug. Do not take any questionable refill medications until you can check with your pharmacist to make sure you have the right medication. If the medication is different, check with your doctor to see if you are supposed to take a different medicine.

Tip #8

While liquid medications in their original packaging are usually not difficult to check, liquid medications in the pharmacy's bottles are harder to check. While you can look up the liquid medication in a PDR and get a description of the liquid as to color or flavor, it is still hard to know if you received the right liquid the first time the prescription is filled. Try having your liquid medications filled by a pharmacist you are familiar with. When refilling liquid medications you can check to establish that the liquid looks and tastes the same as your previous prescription. If you have any questions, make sure you ask before taking the medication.

Tip #9

Making sure you get the right medications in a hospital or nursing home is much harder to do since you do not see original packaging and you may be receiving some medication through an I.V. (receiving drugs through a vein). In addition, you may be sleeping or not feeling well when the medication is given. In these cases, do the best you can and always ask what you are being given and what it is for. Be sure the person who is giving you your medication is aware of any allergies you may have. If possible, have your patient advocate who knows your medical and prescription history find out what drugs have been prescribed for you and why. Your patient advocate can then help verify that you are scheduled to get the right medications. This is especially helpful after surgery when you may be too groggy from anesthesia to ask the right questions. Making sure you are scheduled to receive the right medications is an important step. Your patient advocate should let you know what drugs you should be receiving as soon as you are alert enough to remember the conversation.

Some hospitals and pharmacies are now beginning to use bar code systems and other technology to help prevent drug-dispensing errors. However, not all hospitals are doing this yet, and no system is perfect. Therefore, it's still best to double-check what drugs are being given to you at all times.

Tip #10

If you are filling a prescription for a child, make sure the doctor and pharmacist know the age and weight of the child. Because the size of a child is so varied (at any specific age), the amount of medication given to children is based on their weight. Also, some medications are not given to children until they reach certain ages.

Prescription drugs can and do save lives everyday, but they also can kill if the wrong drug or wrong amount of drug is given. While some of these prescription tips take a little extra time to carry out, it is important to do them. So, be a SMART patient and follow these prescription drug tips. After all, nothing is more important than your health and no one can look out for you as well as you or a loved one can!

Health Care Provider Abbreviations

It is helpful to understand what education/training a health care provider has that is treating you. While you cannot expect to review a resume on all the providers you encounter, you do have the right to ask about their education and training. As mentioned earlier, non-physician health care providers can be a valuable asset during your treatment, but there are situations best addressed only by physicians.

Besides obtaining verbal information from them directly, important clues can be gained by the abbreviations used after their names on business cards, informational brochures, insurance papers, advertisements, etc. Some of the more commonly used abbreviations are listed in Table 3.

Health Care Provider Abbreviations

Table 3

ABBREVIATION	MEANING	THINK
CDA	Certified Dental Assistant	Dental Assistant
D.D.S.	Doctor of Dental Surgery	Dentist
D.M.D.	Doctor of Dental Medicine	Dentist
D.O.	Doctor of Osteopathy	Physician who places more emphasis on the relationship between organs and the musculoskeletal system than a traditional physician does
EMT	Emergency Medical Technician	Ambulance personnel and others who provide emergency care and transport victims to medical facilities
LPN	Licensed Practical Nurse	Nurse who practices under the supervision of a registered nurse
M.D.	Doctor of Medicine	Traditional physician
M.S.	Master of Science or Master of Surgery	Additional training in a particular area
M.T.	Medical Technologist	Performs medical tests
NP	Nurse Practitioner	Registered nurse with advanced training
PA	Physician's Assistant	Practices medicine under the supervision of a physician

ABBREVIATION	MEANING	THINK
PA-C	Certified Physician's Assistant	Practices medicine under the supervision of a physician
PharmD	Doctor of Pharmacy	Pharmacist
Ph.D.	Doctor of Philosophy	Advanced degree in a particular area
PT	Physical Therapist	Therapist helps to restore function to a body after illness or injury
RD	Registered Dietitian	Professional trained in foods and diet management
RDH	Registered Dental Hygienist	Dental hygienist
RN	Registered Nurse	Nurse
RPh	Registered Pharmacist	Pharmacist

In addition to these commonly used abbreviations, you may see other abbreviations or phrases on business cards and other materials. It's common for medical providers to list memberships or affiliations they may have with medical organizations. Examples of this would be using F.A.C.C.P. to indicate being a Fellow of the American College of Chest Physicians or F.A.C.D. to indicate being a Fellow of the American College of Dentists.

Other medical providers may indicate they are Diplomates or Board Certified in certain specialty areas. These medical providers have completed the certification requirements established by a particular medical or dental specialty board. Examples of this would be an orthodontist (dentist who specializes in braces) who is a Diplomate,

American Board of Orthodontics and an orthopedic surgeon (bone, joint, and muscle surgeon) who is a Diplomate, American Board of Orthopedic Surgery.

While all this terminology can be confusing, it's important to know what training the medical providers you see have. When in doubt, ask them about their education and training.

Medical and Dental Specialists

Another helpful tool is to understand what the names of medical and dental specialists mean. This helps you understand that different doctors can help you with different problems. This is especially helpful when you have a serious medical disease or condition that requires you to see many individual specialists. It's not uncommon for the names of specialists to be spoken quickly in your doctor's office so that after you leave the office, you may not remember which doctor does what. As an example, if someone is diagnosed with cancer they may be asked to see an oncologist, a surgeon, and a radiologist. Knowing what areas these doctors specialize in would be helpful in understanding how they would all work together on your behalf.

Medical Specialists

The American Board of Medical Specialties (ABMS) recognizes 25 medical specialties and over 90 subspecialties *(America's Top Doctors*, 2002). The 25 medical specialties recognized by ABMS are:

Allergy and Immunology	Emergency Medicine
Anesthesiology	Family Practice
Colon and Rectal Surgery	Internal Medicine
Dermatology	Medical Genetics

Neurological Surgery

Nuclear Medicine

Obstetrics and Gynecology

Ophthalmology

Orthopaedic Surgery

Otolaryngology

Pathology

Pediatrics

Physical Medicine and Rehabilitation

Plastic Surgery

Preventative Medicine

Psychiatry & Neurology

Radiology

Surgery

Thoracic Surgery

Urology

Listed in Table 4 are some of the more common medical areas and specialists. When you need to know what a specific specialist does, you can look up the name. Again there is no need to memorize these lists. Use them as you need them. (If the specialist you need to see is not on this list you may need to look up the name of the specialist in a medical dictionary.) The list in Table 4 gives the name of the specialty, the name of the doctor (specialist), and a few key words to help you understand what area the specialist helps with. The key words have been taken from definitions in *Mosby's Medical Dictionary*, 6th ed., 2002. You should also keep in mind that there are pediatric specialists for many of the specialties listed below as well. Treating small children is much different than treating grown adults. So there are pediatric neurologists, pediatric endocrinologists, pediatric neurosurgeons, etc. The list includes the 25 specialty areas listed above plus some of the more common names of specialists you may need.

Medical Specialties and Specialists

Table 4

MEDICAL SPECIALTY	SPECIALIST	THINK
Adolescent Medicine	Specialist in Adolescent Medicine	Adolescents
Allergy	Allergist	Allergies
Anesthesiology	Anesthesiologist	Surgery/Pain Management
Cardiology	Cardiologist	Heart
Cardiothoracic Surgery	Cardiothoracic Surgeon	Chest Surgery (Heart/Lung)
Cardiovascular Surgery	Cardiovascular Surgeon	Heart/Blood Vessel Surgery
Colon and Rectal Surgery	Specialist in Colon and Rectal Surgery	Intestine (or Gut) Surgery
Dermatology	Dermatologist	Skin
Emergency Medicine	E.R. Doctor	Accidents/Sudden Illnesses
Endocrinology	Endocrinologist	Hormonal Problems
Family/General Practice	Family Practitioner	General Practice All Ages
Gastroenterology	Gastroenterologist	GI Tract (Mouth to Anus)
Genetics	Geneticist	Genetic/Inherited Problems
Geriatrics	Geriatrician	Elderly Adults
Gynecology	Gynecologist	Female Reproductive/ Breast Health
Hand Surgery	Hand Surgeon	Hand
Hematology	Hematologist	Blood Disorders

MEDICAL SPECIALTY	SPECIALIST	THINK
Immunology	Immunologist	Immune System
Infectious Diseases	Specialist in Infectious Diseases	Communicable Diseases
Internal Medicine	Internist	Internal Organs
Neonatology	Neonatologist	Newborns
Nephrology	Nephrologist	Kidney
Neurology	Neurologist	Brain/Nerve Disorders
Neurosurgery	Neurosurgeon	Brain/Nerve Surgery
Nuclear Medicine	Specialist in Nuclear Medicine	Radioactive Diagnoses/ Treatments
Obstetrics	Obstetrician	Pregnancy/ Childbirth
Oncology	Oncologist	Cancer/ Malignant Diseases
Opthalmology	Opthalmologist	Eye
Orthopaedic Surgery	Orthopaedic Surgeon	Bone/Joint/Muscle Surgery
Orthopedics	Orthopedist	Bones/Joints/Muscles
Otolaryngology	Otolarngologist	Ears/Throat
Otorhinolarngology	Otorhinolarngologist	Ears/Nose/Throat (ENT)
Pathology	Pathologist	Identifies Diseases/ Biopsies
Pediatrics	Pediatrician	Infants/Children
Physical Medicine and Rehabilitation	Physiatrist	Disease/Injury/ Rehabilitation
Plastic Surgery	Plastic Surgeon	Repair/Reconstruct Physical Defects

MEDICAL SPECIALTY	SPECIALIST	THINK
Podiatry	Podiatrist	Feet
Preventative Medicine	Specialist in Preventative Medicine	Prevent Disease
Proctocology	Proctocologist	Colon/Rectum/Anus Disorders
Psychiatry	Psychiatrist	Mental/Mind
Pulmonology	Pulmonogist	Lungs/Respiratory
Radiation Oncology	Radiation Oncologist	Uses Ionizing Radiation to Treat Cancers
Radiology	Radiologist	Reads X-Rays/ Other Tests Diagnosis/Treat with Radioactive Substances
Reproductive Endocrinology	Reproductive Endocrinologist	Infertility/ Reproductive Hormones
Rheumatology	Rheumatologist	Bone/Cartilage/ Connective Tissues Disorders/Arthritis
Sleep Medicine	Specialist in Sleep Medicine	Sleep Disorders
Sports Medicine	Specialist in Sports Medicine	Prevent/Treat Injuries
Surgery	Surgeon	General or Specific Surgery
Thoracic Surgery	Thoracic Surgeon	Chest Surgery
Urology	Urologist	Bladder/Prostate/ Urinary Tract

Dental Specialists

Dentistry is different than medicine with respect to specialists in a couple of ways. First of all, dentistry recognizes fewer dental specialists. The American Dental Association (ADA) recognizes 9 dental specialties (as compared to 25 specialties in medicine and numerous subspecialties). The 9 dental specialties are:

❖ Dental Public Health.

❖ Endodontics.

❖ Oral and Maxillofacial Pathology.

❖ Oral and Maxillofacial Surgery.

❖ Orthodontics and Dentofacial Orthopedics.

❖ Pediatric Dentistry.

❖ Periodontics.

❖ Prosthodontics.

❖ Oral and Maxillofacial Radiology.

The second way dentistry differs from medicine is that general dentists often perform many procedures that dental specialists do. In fact, general dentists may perform whatever procedures he or she feels comfortable providing for their patients. General dentists may not call themselves specialists unless they have completed additional training in a specialty area and are licensed as a specialist.

Table 5 gives the name of the dental specialty, the name of the dental specialist, and a few key words to help you understand what area the specialist helps with. Again, the key words have been taken from definitions in *Mosby's Medical Dictionary*, 6th ed., 2002.

Dental Specialties and Specialists

Table 5

DENTAL SPECIALTY	SPECIALIST	THINK
Dental Public Health	Public Health Dentist	Community Dental Health
Endodontics	Endodontist	Root Canals
Oral and Maxillofacial Pathology	Oral and Maxillofacial Pathologist	Diseases/Studies Biopsies
Oral and Maxillofacial Surgery	Oral Surgeon	Mouth/Jaw Surgery Extract Teeth
Orthodontics and Dentofacial Orthopedics	Orthodontist	Braces/Retainers/ Growth Guidance of Jaws
Pediatric Dentistry	Pedodontist	Children/People with Special Needs
Periodontics	Periodontist	Supporting Tissues of Teeth (Gums/Bone)
Prosthodontics	Prosthodontist	Repairs/Replaces Teeth and Oral Tissues
Oral and Maxillofacial Radiology	Dental Radiologist	Uses X-Ray/ Technology Diagnosis/Treat Diseases

These lists of medical and dental specialists have been included to help you quickly find what area different specialists work in. If you are unable to find the name of a specialist on either the medical or dental lists (or if you need more specific information) then you can consult a medical dictionary at your library or on the Internet.

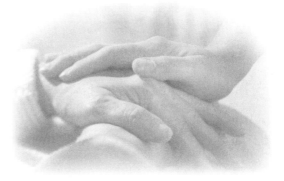

CHAPTER 4

Researching Your Diagnosis

Where do you begin to research your disease or condition? Today there are many excellent resources. Which option or combinations of options you choose will depend on where you live and what is easier for you. While you can start by asking your doctor for information, most doctors do not provide patients with much written information. If you are lucky enough to get written information about a disease or condition from your doctor, it will most likely be a three- or four-page pamphlet. (If you actually get more than this from your doctor, you are very lucky indeed.) If you want more in-depth information about your disease or condition, you or your patient advocate will have to do the research on your own. Thankfully, it's much more easily done than in the past. This chapter discusses some good places to start including:

❖ Associations.

❖ Websites.

❖ Books.

❖ Libraries.

Associations

Associations are available for learning about many specific diseases and a lot of them offer support groups. Associations provide various services to patients and family members alike. They are excellent sources of information and often provide it for free to anyone who requests it (the cost is usually covered by donations). Anyone with access to a telephone can call and get valuable information about their disease or condition without cost. If you are not ready to make the call yourself, you can always have your patient advocate call for information on your behalf. It's a good idea to ask first what support or resources an association may be able to provide in your area. Different associations may be able to provide support or resources to you locally as well as nationally. Associations offer many of the following services:

❖ Help educate the public about diseases
(diagnosis, treatment, prevention, etc.).

❖ Raise valuable research money through donations
(to help treat and fight the disease).

❖ Have a trained staff to answer your questions.

❖ Websites.

❖ Maintain support networks and can often match you
with a support buddy.

❖ Mail out packets of information.

❖ Lead you to other sources of information.

Associations are a great place to start gathering information about your disease or condition. The following is an alphabetical list of associations and organizations for some of the more common medical problems:

ADMINISTRATION ON **AGING**

330 Independence Ave. SW
Washington, D.C. 20201
(202) 619-0724   (800) 677-1116
FAX (202) 260-1012

NATIONAL COUNCIL ON **ALCOHOLISM** AND **DRUG** DEPENDENCE, INC.

12 W 21st St.
New York, NY 10010
(212) 206-6770   (800) NCA-CALL
FAX (212) 645-1690
E-mail: national@ncadd.org
www.ncadd.org

ALZHEIMER'S ASSOCIATION

919 N. Michigan Ave., Suite 1000
Chicago, IL 60611-1676
(312) 335-8700   (800) 272-3900
FAX (312) 335-1110
www.alzgmc.org

ARTHRITIS FOUNDATION

1330 W. Peachtree St.
Atlanta, GA 30309
(404) 872-7100   (800) 283-7800
E-mail: atmail@arthritis.org
www.arthritis.org

ASTHMA AND ALLERGY FOUNDATION OF AMERICA

1223 20th St. NW, Suite 402
Washington, DC 20036
(202) 466-7643   (800) 727-8462
FAX (202) 466-8940
E-mail: info@aafa.org
www.aafa.org

MARCH OF DIMES BIRTH DEFECTS FOUNDATION

1275 Mamaroneck Ave.
White Plains, NY 10605
(914) 997-4526   (888) 663-4637
FAX (914) 997-4537
E-mail: contactus@marchofdimes.com
www.marchofdimes.com

AMERICAN COUNCIL OF THE BLIND

1155 15th St. NW, Suite 1004
Washington, DC 2005
(202) 467-5081   (800) 424-8666
FAX (202) 467-5085
E-mail: info@acb.org
www.acb.org

AMERICAN **CANCER** SOCIETY (ACS) NATIONAL HEADQUARTERS

1599 Clifton Rd.
Atlanta, GA 30329
(404) 320-3333　(404) 329-7648　(800) 227-2345
FAX (404) 325-0230
www.cancer.org

UNITED **CEREBRAL PALSY** ASSOCIATION

1660 L St. NW, Suite 700
Washington, DC 20036
(202) 776-0406　(800) 872-5827
FAX (202) 776-0414
E-mail: national@ucp.org
www.ucp.org

NATIONAL ASSOCIATION OF THE **DEAF**

814 Thayer Street
Silver Spring, MD 20910-4500
(301) 587-1789　TTY (301) 587-1789
FAX (301) 587-1791
E-mail: NADinfor@nad.org
www.nad.org

AMERICAN **DENTAL** ASSOCIATION

211 E. Chicago Ave.
Chicago, IL 60611
(312) 440-2500
www.ada.org

AMERICAN **DIABETES** ASSOCIATION

Attn: National Call Center
1701 N. Beauregard St.
Alexandria, VA 22314
(703) 549-1500   (800) 342-2383
FAX (703) 836-7439
E-mail: customerservice@diabetes.org
www.diabetes.org

NATIONAL **DOWN SYNDROME** SOCIETY

666 Broadway
New York, NY 10012
(212) 460-9330   (800) 221-4602
www.ndss.org

EASTER SEALS

230 W. Monroe St.
Suite #1800
Chicago, IL 60606
(800) 221-6827
E-mail: info@easterseals.com
www.easterseals.com

AMERICAN **GERIATRICS** SOCIETY

The Empire State Building.
350 5th Ave. Suite 801
New York, NY 10118
(212) 308-1414   (800) 247-4779
FAX (212) 832-8646
E-mail: info@americangeriatrics.org

AMERICAN **HEART** ASSOCIATION

7272 Greenville Ave.
Dallas, TX 75231-4596
(214) 373-6300   (800) 242-1793
FAX (214) 706-1341
www.americanheart.org

NATIONAL **HEADACHE** FOUNDATION

428 W St. James Place, 2nd Floor
Chicago, IL 60614-2750
(888) 643-5552
FAX (773) 525-7357
www.headaches.org

NATIONAL **HOSPICE** AND
PALLIATIVE CARE ORGANIZATION

1700 Diagonal Road, Suite 300
Alexandria, VA 22314
(703) 837-1500   (703) 243-5900
(800) 338-8619   (800) 658-8898
FAX (703) 525-5762
E-mail: info@nhpco.org
www.nhpco.org

NATIONAL **KIDNEY** FOUNDATION

30 E 33rd St., Suite 1100
New York, NY 10016
(212) 889-2210   (800) 622-9010
FAX (212) 689-9261
www.kidney.org

AMERICAN **LIVER** FOUNDATION HOME

75 Maiden Ln., Suite 603
New York, NY 10038
(201) 256-2550   (800) 465-4837   (800) 223-0179
FAX (201) 256-3214
E-mail: webmail@liverfoundation.org
www.liverfoundation.org

AMERICAN **LUNG** ASSOCIATION

1740 Broadway
New York, NY 10019-4374
(212) 315-8700   (800) LUNGUSA
FAX (212) 315-8872
E-mail: info@lungusa.org
www.alam.org

AMERICAN **MEDICAL** ASSOCIATION

515 N. State Street
Chicago, IL 60610
(800) 621-8335
www.ama-assn.org

NATIONAL **MENTAL HEALTH** ASSOCIATION

1021 Prince St.
Alexandria, VA 22314-2971
(703) 684-7722   (800) 969-6642
FAX (703) 684-5968
www.nmha.org

MULTIPLE SCLEROSIS ASSOCIATION OF AMERICA

706 Haddonfield Rd.

Cherry Hill, NJ 08002-2652

(609) 488-4500   (800) 532-7667

FAX (856) 661-9797

E-mail: msaa@msaa.com

www.msaa.com

NATIONAL OSTEOPOROSIS FOUNDATION

1232 22nd St. NW

Washington, DC 20037-1292

(202) 223-2226

FAX (202) 223-2237

www.nof.org

AMERICAN PARKINSON'S DISEASE ASSOCIATION

1250 Hylan Blvd., Suite 4-B

Staten Island, NY 10305-1946

(718) 981-8001   (800) 223-2732

FAX (718) 981-4399

www.apdaparkinson.org

AMERICAN ASSOCIATION OF RETIRED PERSONS (AARP)

601 E St. NW

Washington, DC 20049

(202) 434-4277   (800) 424-3410

FAX (202) 434-2320

www.aarp.org

NATIONAL **STROKE** ASSOCIATION

9707 E Easter Lane
Englewood, CO 80112-3747
(303) 649-9299   (800) STROKES
Fax (303) 649-1328
www.stroke.org

While this list is a great starting point for finding associations, you should keep in mind that in today's fast paced world contact information can change rapidly (especially websites). If you are unable to reach an association on this list, you may want to check with telephone information, the Internet, or your library. Similarly, if you are looking for an association for a particular disease or condition and you do not see it here, you can search for one on the Internet (using a search engine) or at your library. There are books that just list names and contact information of associations that can be found at the library. You might ask a librarian. Librarians are great at finding such research information. (Many of the associations and organizations listed above came from an appendix in the back of *Mosby's Medical Dictionary*, 2002.)

Websites

Today many websites offer medical information. While these sites are extremely convenient (you can view them while wearing your bathrobe), you need to be careful about who created and runs the website. It's not difficult to put information on the Internet, but it can difficult to tell if the information is legitimate. Some websites are more reliable than others. Websites run by well-known groups, associations, and universities are more likely to have accurate information than websites run by individuals you don't know.

When researching your disease or condition, use
websites that rely on scientific information that has been
researched. Other websites that offer contact with other
patients are great for support, but you should be careful
about information given there. You need to understand the
difference between fact and someone's opinion. Regardless
of the specific website you use, it's always a good idea
to compare the information from the website with other
information you gather from other sources.

Website addresses (where you find the website) can also change over time. However, many larger associations and groups keep the same address for years. Some health websites you may consider looking at are the websites of the associations listed earlier in this chapter. You can also go to university websites, well-known medical websites, and health websites your local library may be linked to.

A good way to find a large variety of websites providing medical information is to use a search engine website like www.google. com. However, if you use such a search engine you need to narrow your search as much as possible. During a recent search at this website the search words, "websites for human medical information" brought up 704,000 different websites. When the search was narrowed to "layperson websites for human medical information" the search brought up 2250 websites. The second search still brought up a lot of possible websites, but many fewer than the first search. You are better off if you look for a more specific website using a search engine. An example of this would be if you are looking for the website for the University of Michigan Hospital in Ann Arbor, Michigan. Using www.google.com, your search would direct you to the University of Michigan Health System at www.med.umich.edu.

Regardless of which website you choose to look at, it's important to find a website that is written by doctors or organizations that know what they are talking about for the topic you are looking for. Websites written by doctors and organizations tend to have more credibility than websites written by an individual with no official medical training. One of the websites used throughout this book is www.webmd.com. It is a well respected website for medical information. You could also ask your doctor or local librarian if they are familiar with any medical websites that explain things in terms that lay people can understand.

Another source for finding reputable medical websites is the book *Dr. Ian Smith's Guide to Medial Websites* by (you guessed it) Dr. Ian Smith. Dr. Smith is a medical correspondent on NBC's *Today* show. In his book, Dr. Smith gives a rating for each website based on four different criteria. Each website is rated from 1 to 3 (three being the highest rating) in the areas of source, navigation, interactivity, and overall rating. There is a short description of each website. In addition to listing websites alphabetically by medical area or specialty, Dr. Smith also provides a list of the "Top Ten General Medical Websites" (2001). This list includes:

❖ About.com www.about.com

❖ Best Doctors www.bestdoctors.com

❖ HealthAtoZ.com www.healthatoz.com

❖ Healthcommunities.com www.healthcommunities.com

❖ Healthfinder www.healthfinder.gov

❖ InteliHealth   www.intelihealth.com

❖ MedicineNet.com   www.medicinenet.com

❖ National Institute of Health   www.nih.gov

❖ National Library of Medicine   www.nlm.nih.gov

❖ WebMD   www.webmd.com

While Dr. Smith's book lists numerous excellent medical websites, keep in mind that website addresses can change over time.

One other thing to consider is that you do not have to have Internet service at home to have access to the World Wide Web. Besides using a friend's or family member's Internet service, many local libraries have Internet access you can use for free. Many libraries also contract with medical information sources to provide free medical information for their library patrons. Contact your local library to see if they provide a service such as this. Some libraries have a way you can even access this service from home. However, if you only have access to the library's website at the library itself, then you might want to get to the library when they open. Computer terminals tend to fill up fast in some libraries. Reference librarians should also be able to help you find some medical websites to use.

Books

Books are also helpful for learning about specific diseases or conditions. However, because of the length of time it takes to write a book and publish it, some books may not contain the most current information. Associations and websites may be more current. Even so, some reference books are very helpful. Listed below are a sampling of reference books that were found at a local bookstore. The examples are meant to give you a place to start looking. You may find that you like the examples or you may find other books not listed that you like better. Many books can be found under each topic. Regardless of which book you choose, it's good to know where to find (or have) at least one of these reference books under each topic:

Pills (where you look up drug information):

❖ *The Pill Book*, 11th Edition, by Harold M. Silverman (2004)

❖ *The Essential Guide to Prescription Drugs 2004: Everything You Need to Know for Safe Drug Use* by James J. Rybacki (2003)

❖ *The PDR Family Guide to Prescription Drugs*, 9th Edition, by Inc. Medical Economics Company (2002)

PDR® or Physician's Desk Reference (harder to read than a pill book, but has a lot of technical drug information in it):

❖ Updated editions are printed each year. The PDR® for 2005 (for prescription drugs) is the 59th Edition. There are also PDR® books for non-prescription drugs, supplements, and herbal medicines.

Top medical specialists in your country (can help you find the top doctors to see for your problem):

❖ *America's Top Doctors*, 2nd Edition, by Castle Connolly Medical Ltd. (2002)

Common medical diseases and conditions:

❖ *The Merck Manual of Medical Information*, 2nd Edition, by Mark H. Beers (2003)

❖ *American College of Physicians Complete Home Medical Guide*, 2nd Edition, by David R. Goldmann (2003)

❖ *Mayo Clinic Family Health Book*, 3rd Edition, by Mayo Clinic (2003)

Understanding medical tests:

❖ *Mosby's Manual of Diagnostic and Laboratory Tests*, 2ⁿᵈ Edition, by Kathleen Deska Pagana & Timothy J. Pagana (2002)

❖ *The Encyclopedia of Medical Tests*, by Michael B. Brodin (1997)

❖ *Professional Guide to Diagnostic Tests*, by Lippincott Williams & Wilkins (2005)

Medical dictionary (one that is illustrated and has information in the appendices is even better):

❖ *Mosby's Medical Dictionary*, 6ᵗʰ Edition, by Mosby Inc. (2002)

❖ *Dorland's Illustrated Medical Dictionary*, 30ᵗʰ Edition, by W. A. Newman Dorland (2003)

❖ *Stedman's Medical Dictionary*, by Thomas Lathrop Stedman (2000)

❖ *Taber's Cyclopedic Medical Dictionary*, 19ᵗʰ Edition, by Donald Venes, Clayton L. Thomas & Clarence Wilbur Taber (2001)

These books can be purchased at your bookstore or online and some of them may be available at your local library. You might want to consider buying the books you use the most and using your local library for those books used less often. In addition to these general reference books, you may also want to find books on your specific disease or condition. There are many books devoted to individual diseases or conditions.

Finally, having *After the Diagnosis, How to Look Out for Yourself or a Loved One* at your fingertips is always a SMART idea!

Libraries

Libraries are a wonderful source of information when researching your disease or condition. Libraries offer many services:

✤ Books, journals, magazines, tapes.

✤ Internet access (often with medical websites available through the library's own website).

✤ Reference librarians.

When doing research, reference librarians can save you a great deal of time and effort if you take the time to ask them for help. They are acquainted with how to find the latest information on a topic quickly and efficiently.

Remember, part of your tax dollars goes to supporting your local libraries, so you may as well use them. Most libraries offer these services for free (except for damage and late fines). Libraries also offer copy machines so you can take the information home with you without having to write everything down. If you plan on making a lot of copies, you will want to take pocket change with you, as they do charge for using the machine.

Some libraries also specialize in certain areas of information. For example, on university campuses it is not unusual to find libraries associated with different schools. These specialized libraries could include a business library, law library, dental library, medical library, graduate library, undergraduate library, etc. If you are looking for very specific information you might need to go to a certain library to find it. After all, the best place to find dental information is at the dental library.

You may also be able to use the medical library at your local hospital. More and more hospitals are now letting patients use the resources at their own hospital libraries. While you probably cannot check out information there, you may be able to find more specific information that would be hard to find in other places. Hospital libraries tend to have more sophisticated databases for finding medical information when compared to public libraries. It is worth a call to your local hospital to find out what library resources they may be able to offer you.

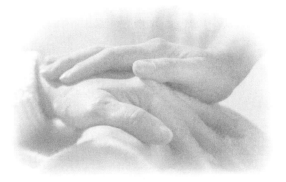

CHAPTER 5

Creating a Plan

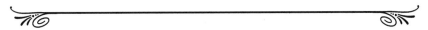

The best thing you can do for yourself or a loved one is to create a plan for dealing with your disease or condition as soon as possible. This may seem like a daunting task, especially if you've just been diagnosed with something serious. For your personal well-being and greater peace of mind, it's important to move forward with a solid plan in place. If you're unable to do this yourself, then ask your patient advocate (see Chapter 1 for selecting a patient advocate) for help. Nothing is more important than your health! Having and using a plan can make a big difference in how your treatment goes and how well your prognosis is. This chapter will deal with:

✧ Continuing with recommended care.

✧ Organizing your care.

✧ Health History form.

❖ Accepting support from health care staff.

❖ Seeking second and third opinions.

❖ Finding top hospitals/care centers and specialists.

❖ What to ask when calling for other opinion appointments.

Continuing with Recommended Care

It is also important to continue with your doctor's recommendations while you are getting your plan together. If your doctor needs you to go through additional testing to determine how far along your disease or condition is, you should do the testing. It is vital that you know if your disease is in the early or advanced stage. How far along your disease is will determine what treatment options are available and what your long-term outcome looks like. While part of you may not want to know, you really need this information in order to give yourself the opportunity for the best treatment and outcome.

If your doctor recommends anything beyond testing, like new medications or surgery, you need to ask him or her how much time you have to make a decision. You need to understand all your options before you start a treatment, medication, or surgery that can permanently change your body or influence later treatment options. For example, if you plan to seek more opinions (and you have time to do so), you may not want to proceed with surgery. The other doctors you see for a second and third opinion may have other ideas on how to treat you. Some doctors may not want to take you on as a patient if you are already in the middle of treatment.

You need to rely on your current doctor's knowledge about how much time you have to decide to proceed with a new treatment. Your doctor should be able to give you an estimate of how long you have to decide. Again, if you are in an emergency situation (heart attack, ruptured hernia, etc.) you may not have much time to decide at all. In other chronic situations (i.e., multiple sclerosis, diabetes) you may have more time to decide. Even with some cancers, there are a few weeks to decide on treatment.

You also need to remember that the time estimate to make decisions your doctor gives you is just that — an estimate. Doctors practice medicine; they do not always have exact answers down to the day. They do their best, but the human body and how it reacts to illnesses can be complicated. What they tell you will be based on their experience with patients in similar situations as yours. Use your time wisely when it comes to the time you have. If your doctor feels you have a week or two to decide, then start researching or ask your patient advocate to begin the research immediately.

> *Be sure to ask your doctor how long you have to decide about treatment without your treatment options or treatment outcome changing significantly or your health being put in jeopardy.*

While we all want time to think and decide about what is best for us or a loved one, don't wait and let a disease get worse before you decide. Take the earliest appointments for testing and consultations that you can. The sooner the testing is finished, the sooner you know what stage of the disease you are in. You need as much information as possible to be able to make good decisions.

A good example of the importance of timing is with cancer treatment. If you know you have cancer and the doctors are confident it's in one area and has not spread, you ought to decide about treatment before it has a chance to spread to other areas of your body. Localized (in one area) cancer is much easier to treat than cancer that has metastasized (spread to other areas of the body). Timing can mean all the difference. The sooner you can make educated decisions, the better.

In summary, proceed with what recommendations your doctor gives you that you are comfortable with and will not change your later treatment options. Use the time estimate to make treatment decisions your doctor gives you to:

✤ Research your disease or condition.

✤ Have your patient advocate research your disease or condition.

✤ Start finding out how to seek second and/or third opinions.

Organizing Your Care

It is very important to be organized about your care because you may have many different doctors, doctor appointments, and testing appointments to keep track of. Keeping track of all of these different things can be confusing unless you have system for organizing all of your medical information. This system can be as simple as having a three-ring binder with dividers in it for keeping all of the similar items together. It's not that different from how medical charts are kept in doctor's offices and hospitals. However, you need to choose a three-ring binder that's large enough. It doesn't take long to fill a binder that's too small. Don't use one that is less than two inches in diameter. Your notebook can be used for your routine medical care or to keep track of a serious illness.

A medical notebook can be helpful to use, but it must contain current and accurate information to be a valuable tool. Appropriate pages should be updated after every medical appointment or event. Updating will help ensure you have the most current information readily available for your health care providers. It will also help you be prepared for any unexpected medical events.

Having all your medical information in one portable notebook will help in many ways:

❖ *You won't have to scramble around the house looking for loose papers.*

❖ *You can take the notebook to your phone when scheduling appointments or speaking with your doctor's office.*

❖ *You can take your notebook to doctor's appointments when you need it.*

While you can modify your notebook to meet specific needs, you should have a divider in the notebook for each of the following sections, in the following order:

1. Calendar — needs to be right up front so you can check dates quickly as you need to schedule appointments. The calendar needs to be big enough to be able to write in appointment times, what the appointments are for, where the appointments are, and a call back phone number. The call back phone number will save you time if you have questions later or need to change an appointment time.

2. Contacts — This section should go right behind your calendar. It will help you more easily locate names, addresses, and phone numbers of medical providers and important people quickly, thus saving you from having to hunt for the same numbers over and over again. You

> *Make a habit of picking up business cards while at your appointments and you'll have the correct spellings of the people you need to speak with.*

might include the following contacts that are involved with your medical care: doctor's offices/medical providers, hospitals, emergency care, relatives, friends, insurance companies, etc.

3. Notes — You need an area where you can write notes. These notes might be written while you are on the telephone, at home, or at the doctor's office. It will be easier to make sense of these notes if you write down the date you are writing them. If your notes involve other people, you should also write down their names. Knowing the name of whom you spoke with, their call back number, and when you spoke to them can be helpful later on if you need to follow up with them again.

4. Medications — You need to keep a current medication list updated and handy. It's an important list to have available for all the health care workers you may be seeing. If you have it all written down, it will save everyone time and you won't forget to tell anyone about any medications you are taking. To help you create your list, you can use the *My Medications* form in Appendix 1. Remember, this list should include the following information:

- ❖ Specific name of medicines you take (including strength and form).

- ❖ How often you take the medicines.

- ❖ When you first started taking the medicines (hours/days/weeks/months or years ago).

❖ Any vitamins, over-the-counter medicines, herbs, or supplements you take.

❖ Allergies you may have (especially drug allergies).

❖ Bad non-allergic reactions to past medications (side effects).

❖ Name and phone number of your pharmacy.

Remember to also use *My New Rx Medication* form (Appendix 1) for all new prescriptions you start.

5. Health history — Keeping a listing of your past and present health history is also a good idea. While you will still have to fill out health history forms when you visit a new doctor's office, having your health history written down will expedite filling out new forms.

An example of a completed *Health History* form is provided on the following pages. When using this form, doctors will ask you more questions about any *yes* answers you may circle. (For photocopying purposes, a blank *Health History* form can be found in Appendix 1.)

The Health History *form should be updated each time there is a significant change in your health. Keeping this form up-to-date may prevent you from forgetting about important facts regarding your health history.*

Health History *(page 1)*

Your Name: <u>IMA Smart Patient</u>

Today's Date: <u>May 2, 2004</u>

Please answer **yes** *or* **no** *to the following questions*
and explain all answers:

1. Are you in good health? <u>Yes, except for thyroid problems</u>

2. Are you currently seeing a physician? If yes, for what reason?
<u>Yes, endocrinologist (for thyroid); had thyroid gland</u>
<u>removed about 6 weeks ago</u>

3. Have you ever been hospitalized? If yes, when and why? <u>Yes</u>
<u>1) Tonsillectomy 1971</u>
<u>2) Arthroscopic surgery on right knee 1994</u>
<u>3) Two children (1998 & 2000)</u>
<u>4) Thyroid removed March 2004</u>

4. Have you ever had surgery? If yes, when and what kind?
<u>Yes, see 1, 2, and 4 under last question</u>

5. Have you ever had a blood transfusion? If yes, when and why? <u>No</u>

Health History *(page 2)*

6. Have you had any change in your health in the past 5 years? _____

Yes, see answers under questions 2 & 3 above

_____

7. Are you allergic to any medication or substance? If yes, provide a specific name (if possible) and list what reaction you had. Penicillin — rash as baby; Clindamycin — rash as adult; Latex allergy — rash, watery eyes, runny nose, and tickle in throat; Allergies to trees, grass, pollen, mold — sinus infections and sore throats

8. Have you had any reaction to a local or general anesthesia? If yes, provide a specific name (if possible) and list what reaction you had.

Spinal anesthesia — spinal headache for 2 weeks (1994)

General anesthesia dizzy for 2 wks after thyroid removed (2004)

9. Do you take any prescription or non-prescription drugs, medicines, or supplements (vitamins/herbs)? If yes, provide specific name, strength, form, how often taken, and when the drug/medicine/supplement was started.

Nexium® 40mg capsule — 1/day before breakfast, started Nov. 2003;

Centrum® multi-vitamin — 1/day with lunch, started years ago;

Tums® XS chewable tablets — 2/day, started after thyroid removal surgery;

Levoxyl® 125mcg tablet — 1/day at bedtime, started after thyroid surgery

10. Did you <u>recently</u> <u>stop</u> taking any prescription or non-prescription drugs, medicines, or pills? If yes, why did you stop?

Propranolol 5 mg (2/day) about 4 wks ago; no longer needed

_____

Health History *(page 3)*

11. **Do you have any of the following diseases, illnesses or medical problems (please circle yes or no):**

yes (no)	Abnormal bleeding	yes (no) Drug abuse
yes (no)	AIDS/ARC	yes (no) Emotional problems
(yes) no	Allergies	(yes) no Endocrine disturbance *thyroid problems*
yes (no)	Anemia	yes (no) Epilepsy
yes (no)	Ankle swelling	yes (no) Excessive thirst
yes (no)	Arthritis	yes (no) Excessive weight loss
yes (no)	Asthma	yes (no) Fainting spells
yes (no)	Auto accident injury	(yes) no Frequent sore throats
yes (no)	Behavorial problems	yes (no) Frequent urination
yes (no)	Birth defects	yes (no) Growth disturbances
yes (no)	Bone disease	yes (no) Hearing problems
yes (no)	Brain illness	yes (no) Heart disease
yes (no)	Breathing problems	(yes) no Heart murmur *no meds needed*
yes (no)	Bruise easily	yes (no) Hemodialysis
yes (no)	Cancer	yes (no) Hemophilia
yes (no)	Chemotherapy	yes (no) Hepatitis
yes (no)	Chest pain	yes (no) Herpes (cold sore)
(yes) no	Chronic pain *muscle aches*	yes (no) High blood pressure
yes (no)	Convulsions	yes (no) HIV
yes (no)	Diabetes	yes (no) Injured during sports
yes (no)	Dizziness	yes (no) Intravenous injections

Health History *(page 4)*

(continued from previous page)

yes (no) Jaundice	yes (no) Rheumatic fever
yes (no) Kidney disease	yes (no) Rickets
yes (no) Liver disease	yes (no) Scarlet fever
(yes) no Low blood pressure	yes (no) Severe headaches
yes (no) Lung disease	yes (no) Shortness of breath
yes (no) Menstrual problems	yes (no) Skin rashes or sores
yes (no) Mental problems	yes (no) Stomach problems
yes (no) Nervous condition	yes (no) Stroke
yes (no) Pacemaker	yes (no) Swollen glands
yes (no) Persistent cough	(yes) no Thyroid disease
yes (no) Persistent diarrhea	yes (no) Tobacco use any form
yes (no) Persistent fever	yes (no) Tuberculosis
(yes) no Persistent tiredness	yes (no) Ulcers
yes (no) Pregnancy	yes (no) Venereal disease
yes (no) Prosthetic heart valve	yes (no) Vision problems
yes (no) Prosthetic joint	yes (no) Vitamin deficiency
yes (no) Radiation therapy	

12. Are their any medical problems that run in your family? If yes, what are they?

Yes, thyroid problems, diabetes, and high blood pressure

_____

_____

_____

_____

6. Questions to ask after the diagnosis — You need a section in your notebook to keep your questions together after you receive a diagnosis. Remember to use the forms in Appendix 1, *Questions to Ask after the Diagnosis, Part I — Initial Questions* and *Questions to Ask after the Diagnosis, Part II — Specific Treatment Recommendations.* This is also a good place to keep the form *What to Ask When Calling for the Other Opinion Appointments* (found in Appendix 1). It is a good idea to keep these papers grouped together by the diagnosis and/or the date they were filled out with the most recent forms being kept in front of older forms.

7. Test results — It's a good idea to get a copy of all your test results whether it's a routine blood test or a test taken due to a serious medical condition. Test results are separated by the type of test taken, the date the test was taken, or by both. Keep similar test results together, making sure to put them in order by date. If you are unsure about what type of test was taken, then filing by date makes the most sense. Keep the most recent test results in front of the older test results so it will be easier to find the most recent ones.

8. Doctor's letters — You should also ask for copies of the letters your doctors send to other doctors or insurance companies. These letters can tell you a lot of things. Often, they will have your diagnosis in them, important test results, and the doctor's recommendations. They may be useful to have when seeking second and third opinions. It also makes sense to file these by date with the most recent letter kept in front of older letters.

9. Billing information — You need a section in the binder to keep all of your medical bills. You may receive medical bills from many different sources, such as doctors' offices, hospitals, laboratories, medical supply companies, etc. If you

keep these bills in order by date of service (most recent in front) you will be able to compare them to the other sections (i.e., test results, insurance) in your notebook more easily.

10. Insurance papers — If you have insurance coverage you will need a section for the insurance papers you will be receiving. If you keep these bills in order by date of service (most recent in front) you will be able to compare them to the other sections (i.e., test results, billing information) in your notebook more easily.

11. Research information — For convenience sake, keep information you have researched about your disease or condition with all your others papers. This information might include website information, articles from magazines or journals, association packets (i.e., packet of requested information from organizations like the American Lung Cancer Association). However, if this section continues to outgrow your binder, it will need to be transferred to another notebook.

12. Care steps — Placing this section in your notebook will give you an area to keep checklists to help make sure you are taking care of the items that need to be done for your medical care. Two checklists can be found later in Chapter 7 that list steps from throughout *After the Diagnosis* and the page numbers these steps can be found on. The *General Care Steps* checklist should be used routinely *before* you encounter a serious diagnosis, while the *After the Diagnosis Care Steps* checklist should be used *after* you have been diagnosed with a problem. These forms were developed as a starting point for you to keep track of the items that need to be considered on your medical journey. You may find that you need to add to these checklists to better fit your particular situation.

13. Other — It is a good idea to have a few extra sections in your notebook for additional information you may want to add later to customize your notebook even more. Planning for extra sections now will just make it easier to add to the notebook later.

It's easier to put this notebook together early on in your diagnosis — or even before you have a serious diagnosis. It's more convenient to keep adding to it as you acquire new pages than to have to sort through 25 to 50 pages of papers all at one time. Periodically, you might want to go through and remove or file certain sections if they are getting too large or becoming unnecessary. This is especially true if you are using your medical notebook for routine appointments and not a serious illness.

If you decide you don't want to take the time to create your own notebook, you can order *My Medical Organizer* by visiting **www.books2helpyou.com**. *My Medical Organizer* is the companion organizer to *After the Diagnosis*. The advantage to using this organizer is that all the initial work has already been done for you! *My Medical Organizer* contains all the divider sections previously described, along with helpful tips. In addition, it contains an Appendix of all the forms used throughout the organizer for easy photocopying. More information is available on page 275 about this organizer.

Purchasing **My Medical Organizer** *allows you to immediately start filling in your medical answers instead of buying/searching for all the necessary items to start your notebook from scratch.*

Accepting Support from Health Care Staff

It is important to remember that there are many other people that can help you create a plan other than your doctor. Among them are nurses, physicians' assistants, medical assistants, medical records personnel, and receptionists. While they will not be able to give you specific medical recommendations in the same way a doctor can, these support people can help you in their own way. They can answer questions you have after seeing the doctor, like: what is the next step, what tests are needed, how to schedule other necessary appointments, how to get copies of medical records, and many other important topics. Health care staff members can also simply provide a friendly smiling face when you need one.

Seeking Second and Third Opinions

While additional opinions may not be needed for a simple problem like an ingrown toenail, they can be invaluable if you have a serious medical problem like lung cancer. If your doctor has determined that you have some time to seek other opinions for a serious medical disease or condition, then you should seek at least a second or even a third opinion. Nothing is more important than your health,

> *It's always a good idea to get acquainted with the staff members of your doctor's office or hospital. Nurses, assistants, and receptionists can be valuable in helping you through your medical journey. They are usually able to spend more time with you than the doctor. It's to your advantage to ask them questions and learn from their experience.*

> *You should be wary of a doctor who tries to sway you away from seeking another opinion when there is time to do so. Doctors worth seeing are not threatened by a patient wanting to seek another opinion. If you perceive the doctor you are seeing as being threatened (by your request for another opinion) then you definitely should get another opinion.*

and seeking second or third opinions will ensure that you are making the right health care decisions.

Nearly everyone knows at least one person who has been misdiagnosed by the first doctor or who may not have received the best recommendations possible. Two case studies are illustrated below, and they show the importance of seeking additional opinions. While the names have been changed to protect the identity of the patients, the situations and facts are true.

CASE STUDY

Jason

The first example pertains to a thirty-year-old man who was having memory trouble and numbness in the big toe of his left foot. Jason was having trouble remembering what he was supposed to be doing at times, and he has had one episode where he couldn't find his way to a known location while driving. His doctor had him take an MRI test of his brain to see if she could find the problem. The results of the MRI came back abnormal. (Jason's MRI results are in Chapter 3 — "How to Read Test Results.") There were many more "spots" (sometimes called UBOs for unidentified bright objects) on the brain scan that weren't normally found on a man of this age. So one Friday evening Jason received a call from his doctor telling him he had multiple sclerosis

(MS) and he needed to see a neurologist. This was a devastating diagnosis, since MS is a lifetime, debilitating disease. After seeing a neurologist, or nerve specialist, the neurologist decided Jason didn't have MS, but instead he had migraines.

Not having severe headaches and still not sure this second diagnosis was correct, Jason decided to seek a third opinion at the neurology clinic of a prominent university hospital. After many tests and appointments, the neurologist did not make a diagnosis at all. The neurologist agreed that the first brain MRI results and other brain MRI results were not what were typically seen in healthy people, but all other tests (blood, spinal fluid, EEG and clinical tests) were normal. Also, Jason's symptoms were not getting any worse. So, rather than label Jason with the wrong diagnosis, this neurologist chose to not make a diagnosis at all. Instead, he referred Jason to another neurologist who specialized in rare neurological conditions.

Jason continued to be followed by this new neurologist (now the fourth opinion) for almost two years. During this time the numbness in Jason's toe disappeared, as did the memory problems. Many tests and appointments later, this neurologist advised Jason to return only if symptoms redeveloped. She never gave Jason a diagnosis either. She agreed that the brain MRI's had been abnormal, but she could find no other abnormalities. Her final recommendation was that there was probably only about a 10 percent chance of Jason developing a serious medical condition later in life. She suggested he get back to living a full normal life.

Ten years later, Jason is doing well. He has not had any more serious memory or numbness problems.

Sometimes doctors don't have all the answers, and we need to respect doctors who can admit this.

In this case study, two doctors gave immediate and wrong diagnoses. Two doctors refused to give a diagnosis because they were not convinced that the evidence and test results supported giving a diagnosis at all. If Jason had not sought the third opinion he might have led a very different life or he might have been prescribed unnecessary medications for a problem he didn't have.

CASE STUDY

Joanne

The second case study is the true story of a woman, sixty-three years old, diagnosed with squamous cell carcinoma of the lung. This story takes place over a much shorter time frame than Jason's, but it also shows the importance of second opinions. Joanne was diagnosed with lung cancer after many years of smoking. There was no question about her diagnosis since it had been determined by a lung biopsy. (Joanne's lung biopsy results can be found in Chapter 3 — "How to Read Test Results.") Additional testing showed that there was only one cancerous tumor; the cancer had not yet spread to other areas of her body. However, because of the location of the cancer, it would eventually kill her if treatment were not done. Her best chance of survival was to have the tumor surgically removed. She also had some significant loss of overall lung function due to the years of smoking.

The first surgeon recommended two surgeries. The first surgery would remove sample lymph nodes in the chest and test them for any evidence of cancer. If the results of the first surgery were good, then a second surgery, about one week later, would be done to remove the actual cancer and part of her right lung. If there was no cancer found in the lymph nodes and Joanne tolerated the anesthesia of the first surgery okay (this was a concern because of her lower level of overall lung function), then the second surgery would be performed to remove the cancer. If the cancer was already in the lymph nodes, then the second surgery would not be done. The first surgeon told her patients did much better if they quit smoking, but he had no other recommendation about preparing her for the surgery.

Joanne's family wanted her to have a second opinion from another surgeon. After confirming with her oncologist, or cancer doctor, that she had enough time to seek another opinion, Joanne sought a second opinion from a surgeon in the cardiovascular surgery department of a prominent university hospital. The surgeon there had a quite different approach to her problem. While he agreed she needed surgery, he wanted to put her through *one surgery, not two*. During this surgery he would sample lymph nodes in the chest first and have them evaluated by a laboratory within the hospital immediately. If the nodes came back cancer free, then the surgeon would remove the cancer and part of her right lung during the same surgery. In addition, the second surgeon wanted her to have an additional lung function test (prior to surgery) to make sure she would have enough lung function remaining after the cancerous part of the lung were removed. If someone does not have enough lung function, they may not even be able to get out of bed.

The second surgeon also asked her to do three things prior to surgery to increase her chances of having successful surgery. He wanted her to quit smoking for good (starting at least three weeks before surgery), walk one to two miles every day, and use a breathing device at home four times a day to give her lungs more exercise. These three recommendations were designed to put Joanne in the best possible health before the surgery. Taking these extra steps would decrease the chances of her ending up in intensive care or having complications after surgery. If Joanne were unwilling or unable to do these three things, the second surgeon would not take her on as a patient.

It didn't take long for Joanne and her family to see that the second surgeon's approach gave her the best chance of successful treatment. Even though the second surgeon's approach was difficult, Joanne followed all three of his recommendations, and she even quit smoking. Joanne underwent surgery with the second surgeon with great success; all of the cancer was removed and none of the lymph nodes showed any signs of cancer! Joanne's recovery went well without any major complications and she continues to be a non-smoker years later.

While both surgeons were both capable of removing the cancer and the lymph nodes, they took quite different approaches to her overall care. The second surgeon prepared her for surgery; the first did not. The second surgeon had her only go through one surgery, not two. And the second surgeon was able to get Joanne to quit smoking when no one else could. If Joanne did not quit smoking, the cancer would have formed in another area for sure. A second opinion made all the difference in the world. The other advantage Joanne had was that she was diagnosed with a slower growing type of lung cancer that was found and treated before it ever had a chance to spread. Joanne has a second chance at life due to finding the cancer in time and finding the right surgeon to treat her.

Because you may not know from the first diagnosis or treatment recommendation if you are seeing the best doctor for your problem, you owe it to yourself to seek other opinions. You may only need one other opinion, or you may end up having to seek third, fourth or even more opinions, depending on what the problem is.

Why are there such differences in opinions among doctors? The truth is that all doctors and specialists have different levels of education, knowledge of the most current information, and opinions.

Additional opinions can either confirm previous opinions or come up with different approaches. If additional opinions simply confirm previous recommendations for your problem, then you can be assured that you would be proceeding with your best treatment option. However, if additional opinions are very different from one another, then you need to use your research information to help you determine who you believe can best help you with your disease or condition. Either way you need to be confident you are in the best hands possible. If you have the time, then seek as many additional opinions as you need to. Finding the right doctor can mean the difference between life and death. The next two sections will show you how to start finding doctors to see for additional opinions.

Finding Top Hospital/Care Centers

Health problems are treated everywhere, but it is in your best interest to find hospitals and care centers that are used to treating patients with your particular disease or condition. Wouldn't you rather be treated at a facility with doctors that do the procedures similar to what you need hundreds of times a year instead of being treated by a doctor who last saw your problem while in medical school?

If you have a common problem that more than likely would be treated the same no matter where you would seek care, then you may be better off seeking treatment closer to home with local medical providers and hospitals. You may receive more individual attention/care in this smaller setting and can save yourself the complications/costs of travel you would encounter if you were treated farther from home. However, if you have a rare condition or disease or if you require more specialized care, you are more likely to benefit from being seen at a top care center. Top care centers are more likely to have seen patients with rare problems and often can provide more specialized care. If you are not sure which option would be better for you and you have time to decide, you might try seeking opinions both locally and at a top care center. The opinions/experience you receive can help you in your decision of where best to have treatment.

Hospitals throughout the United States are ranked by the number of procedures they do and their success rates in different areas of medicine. This is how hospitals become known as top cardiac care centers or top cancer centers in the country.

Listings of top hospital/care centers can be found from various sources, but *U.S. News & World Report* publishes one of the most commonly known and respected listings. Each year this magazine publishes its annual edition of "America's Best Hospitals." Information from their latest edition can be found at your library or on the website at www.usnews.com under "health/best hospitals". For 2004, *U.S. News & World Report* ranked 177 top medical centers in 17 specialty areas of:

Cancer	Ophthalmology
Digestive Disorders	Orthopedics
Ear, Nose & Throat	Pediatrics
Geriatrics	Psychiatry
Gynecology	Rehabilitation
Heart and Heart Surgery	Respiratory Disorders
Hormonal Disorders	Rheumatology
Kidney Disease	Urology
Neurology and Neurosurgery	

When using *U.S. News & World Reports'* website, clicking on any one of these specialty areas will bring up a listing of the top hospitals in the country for that particular specialty area. Besides listing the different hospitals, other information is available, like reputational score, mortality ratio, discharges, number of registered nurses to beds, etc. In another area of their website, *U.S. New & World Report* explains on what criteria the rankings are based.

Contained in their annual edition, *U.S. News & World Report* also has an "Honor Roll" listing of the medical centers. All the medical centers on the Honor Roll ranked high in at least 6 of the 17 Best Hospital specialties. Honor Roll ranking is based on a point system in which hospitals received 2 points for ranking at or near the top in a specialty and 1 point if slightly below that. Below is the Honor Roll listing for 2004:

- ❖ **Johns Hopkins Hospital, Baltimore**
  32 points in 16 specialties

- ❖ **Mayo Clinic, Rochester, Minnesota**
  28 points in 14 specialties

- ❖ **Massachusetts General Hospital, Boston**
  24 points in 13 specialties

- ❖ **Cleveland Clinic**
  24 points in 12 specialties

- ❖ **UCLA Medical Center, Los Angeles**
  23 points in 14 specialties

- ❖ (Tie) **Duke University Medical Center, Durham, N.C.**
  18 points in 10 specialties

- ❖ (Tie) **University of California, San Francisco Medical Center**
  18 points in 10 specialties

- ❖ **Barnes-Jewish Hospital, St. Louis**
  17 points in 11 specialties

❖ (Tie) **New York Presbyterian Hospital**
  17 points in 10 specialties

❖ (Tie) **University of Washington Medical Center, Seattle**
  17 points in 10 specialties

❖ **University of Michigan Medical Center, Ann Arbor**
  13 points in 9 specialties

❖ **Brigham and Women's Hospital, Boston**
  12 points in 8 specialties

❖ **Hospital of the University of Pennsylvania, Philadelphia**
  11 points in 6 specialties

❖ **Stanford Hospital and Clinics, Stanford, California**
  10 points in 7 specialties

Much more specific information about these medical centers is available in the annual magazine edition of "America's Best Hospitals" or at the *U.S. News & World Reports'* website. Clicking on any one of these medical centers within the website will bring up more information about each center including a listing of each center's ranking for the different specialties. This will allow you to know how each medical center ranked for a particular specialty you may be interested in.

While rankings of medical centers can be very helpful they also need to be viewed with a little caution. Some medical centers/hospitals take such rankings very seriously and they want to continue to be ranked as high as possible. While no one likes to admit it, medical providers at some hospitals may be more likely to treat patients who have more favorable prognoses (outcomes) and less likely to treat more difficult cases who would have less favorable prognoses (outcomes). Selecting patients with better chances for success from the beginning would artificially improve a medical center's success statistics and result in higher rankings compared to other medical centers. Similarly, other medical centers/hospitals that do not place such emphasis on their success statistics may have medical providers who are more willing to take on the tougher cases. In other words, some medical centers/hospitals may provide excellent care, but not be a top ranked medical center/hospital because of their willingness to treat everyone, even the tough cases.

For these reasons, if you have a rare problem or require specialized care you should look at top hospital/care centers official listings, but you should also ask your current medical providers what are the best hospital/care centers for your particular problem. They may be able to provide additional information about specific hospital/care centers to help you find the best place for your care. Friends or family members may also know of top hospital/care centers for specific problems.

If you choose to visit a medical facility (like a top center/ hospital) or medical provider (like a top specialist) you have not been to before, make sure the medical facility/medical provider will accept your specific insurance coverage. You should check with the facility's biller, the provider's biller, and your own insurance company. It is not unusual for facilities like hospitals and the doctors who work there to bill you separately. It is possible to go to a hospital (in-network) and be treated by a doctor there (out-of-network) and then have differences in how your insurance company makes payment to them. (See Chapter 6 for a discussion of in-network and out-of-network charges.) If you do not take the time to understand what payments the facility will accept from your insurance and what payments are expected from you, you could end up with large unexpected medical bills!

Finding Top Specialists

Finding a top specialist in the area you need is even more important than which hospital you end up in. If you have a serious disease or problem, it is in your best interest to be treated by the best doctor you can find. Top specialists are often found at the best medical centers. Top specialists in the United States, like hospitals, are also ranked by the number of procedures they do and their success rates in different areas of medicine. A good source for finding top specialists is a book titled *America's Top Doctors*, published by Castle Connolly, and it lists the top doctors by geographic area in the country (U.S.) and by specialty. This book lists doctors in the following specialties:

Adolescent Medicine

Allergy & Immunology

Cardiology

Child Neurology

Clinical Genetics

Colon & Rectal Surgery

Dermatology

Endocrinology, Diabetes & Metabolism

Gastroenterology

Geriatric Medicine

Gynecologic Oncology

Hand Surgery

Hematology & Medical Oncology

Infectious Disease

Internal Medicine

Maternal & Fetal Medicine

Neonatal-Perinatal Medicine

Nephrology

Neurology

Neurological Surgery

Neurology

Nuclear Medicine

Obstetrics/Gynecology

Ophthalmology

Orthopaedic Surgery

Otolaryngology

Pain Management

Pathology

Pediatrics

Physical Medicine & Rehabilitation

Plastic Surgery

Psychiatry

Pulmonology

Radiation Oncology

Radiology

Reproductive Endocrinology

Rheumatology

Sports Medicine

Surgery

Thoracic Surgery

Urology

Vascular Surgery (General)

This book also contains a great deal of other helpful information in the introduction on making the most out of seeing top specialists. As well, Castle Connelly publishes regional books for top doctors for the New York metropolitan area and the Chicago metropolitan area. More information can be found on their website at www.americastopdoctors.com.

In addition to looking at official listings, you should always ask your physicians which specialists they recommend for your particular problem. Friends or family members may also know of top specialists meant for specific problems.

What to Ask When Calling for Other Opinion Appointments

The names for seeking other opinions may come from your doctor, relatives, friends, or coworkers. Ask everyone you know. Someone may recommend an excellent specialist to see for your particular disease or condition. Additional names could come from your research of top hospitals and specialists. Sometimes these two lists may even contain a few of the same people. Wherever possible, have *specific names*. This is especially helpful when you are calling a large hospital or care center. If you don't have a specific name in mind, you will probably end up seeing the "newer" doctor who has more appointment time available, but less experience.

Once you have one or more names and phone numbers with which to seek other opinions, you need to know what questions to ask. Knowing this will save you precious time and energy. While your particular situation may require some modification of these suggestions, the following questions will give you a good place to start. When you call to ask these questions, write down the date and time you called and whom you spoke with. This way, if there are ever any questions about what was said, you will be able to remember the person's name.

1. Is the doctor I want to see accepting new patients?

If the answer is no, you will have try another name on your list. If the answer is yes, you need to explain why you are calling and find out if there is a reason why the doctor might not take you on as a patient. Doctors turn down seeing new patients for a variety of reasons. Sometimes they choose not to see a new patient if the patient has already begun certain treatments (i.e., participating in a clinical trial). Another reason would be an obstetrician (a doctor who delivers babies) that decides not to see a woman who is already eight months pregnant. In this case, the doctor may not want to undertake another doctor's management plan that far along in pregnancy since he or she wasn't able to guide the mother on proper prenatal care from the beginning of the pregnancy.

2. Does the doctor accept my insurance?

With the high cost of medical care this is an important question and needs to be asked early on in your conversation. You can ask this question to the receptionist who answers the phone, but you might have to speak with the person who directly handles the billing for the office. If the doctor does accept your insurance, then ask what fees you may be responsible for, especially for the beginning appointments. If the doctor does not accept your insurance, you have one of two options. The first is to find another doctor. The second option is to be responsible for all the treatment fees on your own. Asking up front what fees you would be expected to pay can save both you and the office a great deal of time. There is no use starting a relationship with a doctor you don't intend to see in the long run.

3. How long will I have to wait for the first appointment?

This is always an important question to ask and the answer can vary greatly depending on your disease or condition and in which area of medicine the doctor practices. If you have a non-life-threatening problem and you need to see a dermatologist, you may not be able to get an appointment as a new patient for six to twelve weeks or longer. However, if you find out you have cancer and call an oncologist's office they know to see you as soon as possible (usually within a few days). How long you have to wait for an appointment can also vary depending on who is calling. Sometimes you can get an earlier appointment by having your current doctor's office call for you. A doctor's office will often call a specialist's office and explain the need for you to be seen as soon as possible if you have a serious medical condition.

> *Keep in mind that if you have a serious problem you should take the first available appointment offered to you. Do not waste an opportunity to be seen sooner because you don't like the appointment time or you cannot make a decision. If you do not take the appointment, the next person will! You can always call back later to change an appointment.*

If the person you really want to see is booked for several weeks and you have a serious medical condition, then ask your current doctor if you will be harmed in any way by waiting for this other opinion appointment. If the answer is no, then keep the appointment, but ask if you can be placed on a waiting list in the event there is a cancellation. Some offices don't have waiting lists and may ask you to call on a daily basis to see if there have been any cancellations. Either way, if you want to be seen as soon as possible, be willing to take an appointment any day and any time. On the other hand, if the answer from your current doctor is that you should not wait weeks for this additional opinion, then ask your current doctor if he or she would call and see if you could be seen sooner. If you cannot be seen sooner even after your doctor has called for you, then you need to try the next doctor on your list.

The next doctor on your list may be in a totally different office or you might consider seeing the *newer* doctor in the same practice as the doctor you are unable to see quickly. It is often easier to get an appointment quickly with a *newer* doctor since they don't have as many patients to see as more established doctors do. While the *newer* doctor will not have the same experience as your first choice doctor, they should be able to consult with the other doctor(s) in their practice (the doctor you originally wanted to see). Your current doctor can help you decide who should be the next doctor on your list to try for an appointment.

If you are trying to schedule an appointment with a nationally known doctor, you may have to wait a while — or you may be pleasantly surprised and be able to be seen right away. You won't know until you call!

4. What medical records does the office need and when do they need them?

In some situations you may not be able to make an appointment to see a doctor until after you forward copies of your medical records to his or her office. Some offices will not schedule an appointment until all the necessary information is in their hands. While forwarding your medical information is an extra step, it gives the doctor an opportunity to know much more about you before an appointment is made. The doctor can make sure he or she can help you in the first place and he or she can begin to develop a plan before you arrive. In other situations, you can bring your medical records with you to the first appointment. Either way, just make sure that the doctor's office has whatever information they need when they need it. You do not want your treatment delayed because they are missing a test result.

The first step is to write down a list of exactly what information the office wants available. Sometimes this can simply be the referral slip you received from your doctor. Other times the office may need a copy of every test result, letter, biopsy, and report you have relating to your current problem. They may also request the actual radiographs (x-ray films) or biopsy slides. Make sure you write down everything they are asking for, and whom you spoke to and when, in case you have any questions later on.

Today, many radiology departments will (upon your request) provide copies of your actual film studies for you to keep and take with you to future doctor appointments. Some radiology departments

It is always a good idea when contacting a new office to ask if they can send you their first appointment paperwork ahead of time (by mail or fax). This gives you the opportunity to fill out their paperwork (usually a health history and payment/insurance forms) before your appointment. This extra step gives you more time to be complete and also can help you feel less rushed the day of your appointment. Some offices routinely send paperwork ahead of time, while others will do so only upon request. If you do receive the paperwork ahead of time, you must remember to bring the completed forms to your appointment.

now even provide all of the film studies in digital format conveniently contained on a compact disc (CD). Other radiology departments may only loan out your film studies and ask that you return them when you are finished with them. You need to ask at your specific radiology department what options you have for using/keeping your radiology test results.

Once you know what medical information needs to be forwarded, then you or your patient advocate needs to get all the information forwarded as soon as possible. The fastest way today to get written information to its destination is to fax it. Fax what information you may have or ask your current doctor's office to fax it for you. Other material information, like radiographs or pathology slides, may need to picked-up from offices or hospital record rooms and hand carried by you or sent by medical courier to the new office. Try to do this as quickly as possible and always verify that all your needed medical information arrived safely at the doctor's office. The sooner the office has your information, the sooner you can be seen.

5. Is any additional testing needed before I am seen?

An office may not be able to answer this question until they have had a chance to review your medical information. However, asking this question can save you time. For example, if your last chest radiograph was three months ago and they want another one taken close to your appointment, then coordinate arrangements with their office to have it done. You also need to make sure any needed reports/films will be sent to their office before your appointment time. In this way the doctor can have the most recent information about you as possible.

6. How long can I expect to be at the first appointment?

Asking this question ahead of time can prevent any surprises at this first appointment. You do not want to find out you are scheduled for a two-hour appointment when you had only planned on being there for fifteen minutes. Similarly, even when you are given an estimated appointment length, plan for extra time. Unexpected situations do come up that put a medical office behind schedule. Also if you plan to see a nationally recognized doctor or top specialist, be prepared to wait patiently for your turn to see him or her. While no one wants to wait, you may have to wait for long periods of time to see the best. If a top doctor can save your life, then he or she will be well worth waiting for.

7. How do I get there?

It's always a good idea to know where you are going so you can arrive at your appointment on time. Some offices will give you verbal directions, while other offices, especially medical centers, will send you a map along with a letter confirming your appointment time. If you require wheelchair access or do not like to ride elevators, then make sure you ask about how to solve these issues as well. It is also a good idea to plan on arriving fifteen minutes early to your appointment. This will allow extra time for filling out paperwork (if needed) or provide an extra cushion of time in case you get caught in traffic or become lost on the way to a new office. Planning for a little extra time before your appointment will help you arrive ready for your actual appointment time.

Finally, ask any questions that you want answered or might be special for your particular situation. Perhaps you have special needs that must be addressed for you to go to a particular office or facility. An example of this would be if you have a latex allergy and you need to seek care from a place that understands your allergy and your need to avoid latex. Another example would be if you are deaf and you need someone to translate for you using sign language. Does the facility have a sign language translator, or do you need to bring someone with you?

Taking the time to ask questions will save both you and the new doctor's office time and energy in the long run. Posing the right questions may also help to speed up how quickly you are seen.

The questions we've covered are summarized for you in the *What to Ask When Calling for the Other Opinion Appointments* form. A completed example of this form is provided on the next two pages. (For photocopying purposes, a blank *What to Ask When Calling for the Other Opinion Appointments* form can be found in Appendix 1.)

Securing an appointment to see a specialist or a top doctor is a great step forward, but you also need to remember what questions to ask so you can get the most benefit from this appointment. Don't forget to use the forms from Chapter 2, found in Appendix 1, Questions to Ask after the Diagnosis, Part I — Initial Questions *and* Questions to Ask after the Diagnosis, Part II — Specific Treatment Recommendations. *Bring these forms with you to all your appointments. They not only provide important facts and history about your diagnosis, but they also allow room for new information to be collected as well.*

What to Ask When Calling for
the Other Opinion Appointments *(page 1)*

Your Name: _IMA Smart Patient_

Doctor's Name: _Thyroid Genius, M.D._

Doctor's Phone #: _734-936-6000_

Who You Spoke With: _Aleigha_

Today's Date: _January 2, 2004_

1. Is the doctor accepting new patients?

(Yes)   No

2. Does the doctor accept your insurance?

(Yes)   No

3. How long will I have to wait for the first appointment?

_____Days   _~3_ Weeks   _____Months

(Is your doctor comfortable with you waiting this long to be seen? (Yes) No)

4. What medical records does the office need? When are they needed?

_X_ Blood reports   ____ Doctor's referral(s) and/or letter(s)

____ X-rays reports   ____ Actual x-ray films

_X_ CAT scan reports   _X_ Actual CAT scan films

____ MRI scan reports   ____ Actual MRI scan films

_X_ Ultrasound reports   _X_ Actual ultrasound films

_X_ Biopsy reports   _X_ Pathology slides needed (from biopsy)

____ Health history form (if sent to you by the new office/completed by you)

____ Payment/Insurance form (if sent to you by the new office/completed by you)

What to Ask When Calling for
the Other Opinion Appointments *(page 2)*

____Other items needed _____

_____

_____

When are records needed?   ASAP (before appointment is made)?

Or bring all items to first appointment?

5. Is any additional testing needed before you are seen?

No   If Yes, then what _____

_____

6. How long can I expect to be at the first appointment?

_____Minutes   2   Hours

7. Questions about location, directions or access to the building?

Will a map be sent?   Yes   No   If No, then how will I get there?

_____

_____

Is the office or facility handicap accessible?   Yes   No

8. Questions for your particular situation: _____

Is the office latex safe — yes

Are powdered latex gloves used for any patients — no

_____

_____

_____

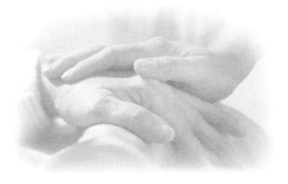

CHAPTER 6

Payments and Insurance

Medical payments and insurance coverage have become a complicated issue. Long gone are the days when medical services were paid for strictly on a cash basis. Today, payments are made by cash, check, credit cards, and through insurance company payments. People have medical and dental insurance coverage through many different insurance companies and each has their own policies and terms, often determined by the employer. Sometimes an individual may be covered by multiple insurance plans as well. Above and beyond insurance coverage, people can contribute to other accounts (e.g., flexible spending accounts or medical savings accounts) offered through their employer, using pre-tax dollars, to help pay for medical and dental expenses.

In addition, medical and dental fees can vary greatly for procedures and services performed in different settings and different parts of the country. Just as movie ticket prices or gasoline prices vary, depending on what source you purchase them from and where they are geographically located, so can medical and dental fees vary from different sources and geographic locations. As an example, these differences can be seen by someone purchasing orthodontic braces. The person seeking orthodontic treatment will find a difference in price for the service whether they decide to be treated at a dental school clinic or in an exclusive private orthodontic practice. The dental school fee for braces is usually significantly less than the fee for braces found in private practice. (Having said this, receiving orthodontic treatment in a dental school will require more time for each appointment since treatment is being delivered in a teaching setting.) Similarly, the fee for braces from a general dentist may be less than the fee for braces from an orthodontic specialist. Also, the fee for the same treatment for braces can be more if treatment is sought in a geographically wealthy area vs. an area less well off financially. While all of these differences may not seem fair, they are a reality.

For these reasons, it's impossible to discuss exact details about your specific medical payments or insurance coverage. However, this chapter will give you helpful information so you can better understand your particular situation. Part of what makes payments, contributions, and insurance coverage seem so confusing is the use of so many different technical terms. If you don't understand the terms used to explain your benefits, you cannot understand your coverage.

This chapter is designed as a reference tool. You should always ask your doctor's office or insurance company for specific information regarding your payments and insurance benefits.

The main sections of this chapter include:

✤ Payment and insurance definitions.

✤ Payment and insurance tips.

✤ Insurance Information form.

Payment and Insurance Definitions

Listed below are definitions to help you understand the right questions to ask for your particular situation.

Claim

A *claim* is defined as "a demand for payment from a provider for care that has been rendered". (*Mosby's Medical Dictionary*, 2002)

COBRA (Consolidated Omnibus Reconciliation Act)

COBRA stand for "legislation that provides for limited continuation of health coverage for individuals and families at the individual's own expense when the individual terminates employment from an organization that provides health insurance. The law applies only to organizations with a specified number of employees." (*Mosby's Medical Dictionary*, 2002)

Coinsurance

Coinsurance is defined as "a form of medical cost sharing in a health insurance plan that requires an insured person to pay a stated percentage of medical expenses after the deductible amount, if any, was paid.

❖ Once any deductible amount and coinsurance are paid, the insurer is responsible for the rest of the reimbursement for covered benefits up to allowed charges: the individual could also be responsible for any charges in excess of what the insurer determines to be 'usual, customary and reasonable'.

❖ Coinsurance rates may differ if services are received from an approved provider (i.e., a provider with whom the insurer has a contract or an agreement specifying payment levels and other contract requirements) or if received by providers not on the approved list.

✤ In addition to overall coinsurance rates, rates may also differ for different types of services." (Website of the USA Federal Government, 2004 — see References)

An example of coinsurance would be you having to pay 15 percent of a bill for blood testing after your insurance paid 85 percent of the bill. This example assumes that you had already paid your deductible for the year.

Conventional Indemnity Plan/Traditional Plan

A *conventional indemnity plan* is defined as "an indemnity plan that allows the participant the choice of any provider without effect on reimbursement. These plans reimburse the patient and/or provider as expenses are incurred." (Website of the USA Federal Government, 2004 — see References)

Copayment

A *copayment* is defined as "a form of medical cost sharing in a health insurance plan that requires an insured person to pay a fixed dollar amount when a medical service is received. The insurer is responsible for the rest of the reimbursement.

✤ There may be separate copayments for different services.

✤ Some plans require that a deductible first be met for some specific services before a copayment applies." (Website of the USA Federal Government, 2004 — see References)

An example of a copayment is a flat rate you pay for an office visit each time you visit a physician's office. This flat rate can be a different amount depending on what type of doctor you are seeing: a primary physician (internist, pediatrician, etc.) or a specialist (surgeon, cardiologist, etc.).

Deductible (Individual/Family)

Deductible is defined as "a fixed dollar amount during the benefit period (usually a year) that an insured person pays before the insurer starts to make payments for covered medical services. Plans may have both per individual and family deductibles.

❖ Some plans may have separate deductibles for specific services. For example, a plan may have a hospitalization deductible per admission.

❖ Deductibles may differ if services are received from an approved provider or if received from providers not on the approved list." (Website of the USA Federal Government, 2004 — see References)

Dependent

For purposes of insurance terms, *dependent* refers to a person who has insurance benefits because another person is enrolled in the insurance plan. Dependent usually refers to children and spouses of an enrollee.

Eligibility

Eligibility is defined as "entitlement of an individual to receive services based on that individual's enrollment in a health care plan". (*Mosby's Medical Dictionary*, 2002)

Enrollee/Member

An *enrollee* or *member* is defined as "an individual who has signed up to receive health care under a particular type of plan". (*Mosby's Medical Dictionary*, 2002)

Exclusive Provider Organization (EPO)

An *exclusive provider organization* is defined as "a more restrictive type of preferred provider organization plan under which employees must use providers from the specified network of physicians and hospitals to receive coverage; there is no coverage for care received from a non-network provider except in an emergency situation". (Website of the USA Federal Government, 2004 — see References)

Explanation of Benefits (EOB)

An *explanation of benefits* is, as the name implies, a statement from the insurance company explaining what benefits have been paid out for what services. EOBs are often sent by mail, but many companies also offer viewing of them online at the company's website. The EOB will explain, for a particular service date, items such as what charges were submitted by a provider (doctor's office, laboratory, hospital, etc.), on behalf of which patient; what copay is due; whether or not any of the charges were applied to a deductible; at what percentage the claim was paid; how much the insurance company paid the provider; and how much, if any, the patient or parent is responsible for paying.

It is important to read the EOB carefully in order to be sure that claims are being processed according to your actual benefits. Mistakes can be made during claim processing. It is to your benefit to double check to make sure you understand and agree with the EOB.

Flexible Spending Account (FSA)

A *flexible spending account* is defined as "accounts offered and administered by employers that provide a way for employees to set aside, out of their paycheck, pretax dollars to pay for the employee's share of insurance premiums or medical expenses not covered by the employer's health plan. The employer may also make contributions to an FSA. Typically, benefits or cash must be used within the given benefit year or the employee loses the money. Flexible spending accounts can also be provided to cover child care expenses, but those accounts must be established separately from medical FSAs." (Website of the USA Federal Government, 2004 — see References)

Flexible Benefits Plan (Cafeteria Plan)

A *flexible benefits plan* is defined as "a benefit program under Section 125 of the Internal Revenue Code that offers employees a choice between permissible taxable benefits, including cash, and nontaxable benefits such as life and health insurance, vacations, retirement plans, and child care. Although a common core of benefits may be required, the employee can determine how his or her remaining benefit dollars are to be allocated for each type of benefit from the total amount promised by the employer. Sometimes employee contributions may be made for additional coverage." (Website of the USA Federal Government, 2004 — see References)

Group Number

The *group number* is a number used for processing claims. It helps identify what group policy the enrollee belongs to. The insurance company uses a group number together with the member number to determine what benefits the enrollee is entitled to. It is also used during all claim processing.

Health Maintenance Organization (HMO)

A *health maintenance organization* is defined as "a type of group health care practice that provides basic and supplemental health maintenance and treatment services to voluntary enrollees who prepay a fixed periodic fee that is set without regard to the amount or kind of services received. In addition to diagnostic and treatment services, including hospitalization and surgery, an HMO often offers supplemental services, such as dental, mental, and eye care, and pre-scription drugs". (*Mosby's Medical Dictionary*, 2002)

Participating in this type of insurance plan usually means you will pay less yourself for services since you pay a fixed periodic fee whether you use the services or not, but you have less control over the care received. You must seek care at participating facilities with participating physicians. It can also be more difficult to see a special-ist. Oftentimes a primary physician must refer you to the specialist or the specialist's fees will not be covered.

Indemnity Plan

An *indemnity plan* is defined as "a type of medical plan that reim-burses the patient and /or provider as expenses are incurred". (Website of the USA Federal Government, 2004 — see References)

In-Network/Participating

The terms *in-network* or *participating* refer to the group of selected health care providers, such as hospitals and physicians, servicing patients of a particular health care plan. In-network providers have signed a contract to provide services to an insurance plan's members, usually at agreed upon service rates. Some health care plans require its enrollees to see only in-network providers, except for emergen-cies, while other health care plans allow its enrollees to seek care out-of-network, but at increased costs to the enrollee.

Lifetime Maximum Benefit (Maximum Plan Dollar Limit)

Maximum plan dollar limit is defined as "the maximum amount payable by the insurer for covered expenses for the insured and each covered dependent while covered under the health plan.

✧ Plans can have a yearly and/or a lifetime maximum dollar limit.

✧ The most typical of maximums is a lifetime amount of

$1 million per individual." (Website of the USA Federal Government, 2004 — see References)

There can be separate lifetime maximum dollar limits for services used in-network and those used out-of-network.

Managed Care Plans

"*Managed care plans* generally provide comprehensive health services to their members, and offer financial incentives for patients to use the providers who belong to the plan. Examples of managed care plans include:

❖ Health maintenance organizations (HMOs).

❖ Preferred provider organizations (PPOs).

❖ Exclusive provider organizations (EPOs).

❖ Point of service plans (POSs)." (Website of the USA Federal Government, 2004 — see References.)

Medicaid

Medicaid is defined as, "A U.S. federally funded state operated program of medical assistance to people with low incomes, authorized by Title XIX of the Social Security Act. Under broad federal guidelines the individual states determine benefits, eligibility, rates of payment, and methods of administration." (*Mosby's Medical Dictionary*, 2002)

Medical Savings Accounts (MSA)

A *medical savings account* is defined as "savings accounts designated for out-of-pocket medical expenses. In an MSA, employers and individuals are allowed to contribute to a savings account on a pre-tax basis and carry over the unused funds at the end of the year. One major difference between a Flexible Spending Account (FSA) and a Medical Savings Account (MSA) is the ability under an MSA to carry over the unused funds for use in a future year, instead of losing unused funds at the end of the year. Most MSAs allow unused balances and earnings to accumulate. Unlike FSAs, most MSAs are combined with a high deductible or catastrophic health insurance plan." (Website of the USA Federal Government, 2004 — see References)

Medicare

Medicare is defined as "a federally funded national health insurance program in the United States for people over 65 years of age. The program is administered in two parts. Part A provides basic protection against costs of medical, surgical, and psychiatric hospital care. Part B is a voluntary medical insurance program financed in part from federal funds and in part from premiums contributed by enrollees. Medicare enrollment is offered to people 65 years of age or older who are entitled to receive Social Security or railroad retirement benefits. Other people above 65 years of age, such as federal employees and aliens, may not be eligible. Medicare was authorized by Title XVIII of the Social Security Act of 1965." (*Mosby's Medical Dictionary*, 2002)

Member (see Enrollee)

Member ID

The *member ID* number is the number used by insurance companies to identify enrollees. This number is often the enrollee's social security number. However, for privacy and security reasons, insurance companies are moving towards adding a few extra numbers to the social security number or assigning a totally different number (other than SS#) to each enrollee.

Negotiated Amount (Negotiated Fee, Charge or Rate)

The *negotiated fee* is a fixed dollar amount for a covered service that is previously agreed upon between the insurance company and the provider of services (physician, hospital, etc.). It is often used in managed insurance plans like the PPO. When negotiated fees are used, the provider agrees to accept the amount of the negotiated fee as payment in full for a service. The patient is not responsible for any amount charged over the negotiated fee, as long as the provider is an in-network provider.

Network Providers

Network providers are the health care providers, such as hospitals and physicians, who are part of a group of selected providers to provide services for a particular health care plan. Some health care plans require its enrollees to see only in-network providers (except for emergencies), while other health care plans allow its enrollees to seek care out-of-network, but at increased costs to the enrollee.

Non-Participating Provider (see Out-of-Network Provider)

Out-of-Network/Out-of-Plan Services

Out-of-network services are defined as "services given to a patient by a provider outside the managed care system. The patient may be responsible for a larger co-payment than if the services were received within the plan." (*Mosby's Medical Dictionary*, 2002)

Out-of-Network Providers

Out-of-network providers are the health care providers, such as hospitals and physicians, who are *not* part of a group of selected providers to provide services for a particular health care plan. Out-of-network providers have not signed a contract to provide services to an insurance plan's members. Some health care plans require its enrollees to see only in-network providers (except for emergencies), while other health care plans allow its enrollees to seek care out-of-network, but at increased costs to the enrollee.

Out-of-Pocket Limit

An *out-of-pocket* limit is defined as "the maximum dollar amount a group member is required to pay out of pocket during a year. Until this maximum is met, the group member shares in the cost of covered expenses. After the maximum is reached, the insurance carrier pays all covered expenses, often up to a lifetime maximum." (Website of the USA Federal Government, 2004 — see References)

There can be separate individual and family out-of-pocket limits.

Point-of-Service (POS) Plan

A *point-of service plan* is defined as "an HMO/PPO hybrid; sometimes referred to as an open-ended HMO when offered by an HMO. POS plans resemble HMOs for in-network services. Services received outside of the network are usually reimbursed in a manner similar to conventional indemnity plans (e.g., provider reimbursement based on a fee schedule or usual, customary and reasonable charges)." (Website of the USA Federal Government, 2004 — see References)

Preexisting Condition

A *preexisting condition* is defined as "any injury, disease, or disability that may have occurred at some time in the past and may predispose an individual to limited health in the future". (*Mosby's Medical Dictionary*, 2002)

Depending on how an insurance policy is written, insurance companies may choose to exclude some benefits for individuals with preexisting conditions.

Preferred Provider Organization (PPO)

A *preferred provider organization* is defined as "an indemnity plan where coverage is provided to participants through a network of selected health care providers (such as hospitals and physicians).

The enrollees may go outside the network, but would incur larger costs in the form of higher deductibles, higher coinsurance rates, or non-discounted charges from the providers." (Website of the USA Federal Government, 2004 — see References)

When you have PPO insurance you are encouraged to use services with the network. If you choose to go outside the network of providers, you will end up paying more for service.

Pre-Admission Certification

Pre-admission certification is defined as "an authorization for hospital admission given by a health care provider to a group member prior to their hospitalization. Failure to obtain a readmission certification in non-emergency situations reduces or eliminates the health care provider's obligation to pay for services rendered." (Website of the USA Federal Government, 2004 — see References)

Pre-Authorization

Pre-authorization is the term used for submitting information to an insurance company regarding a planned medical or dental procedure or service before the procedure or service actually takes place. The information is submitted prior to being done so the provider (i.e., doctor, laboratory, or hospital) and enrollee will know how much the insurance company will pay when the procedure or service is actually completed (assuming there is no change in insurance coverage due to change in job, etc.).

Premium

Premium is defined as "agreed upon fees paid for coverage of medical benefits for a defined benefit period. Premiums can be paid by employers, union, employees, or shared by both the insured individual and the plan sponsor." (Website of the USA Federal Government, 2004 — see References)

Primary Care Physician (PCP)

Primary care physician is defined as "a physician who serves as a group member's primary contact within the health plan. In a managed care plan, the primary care physician provides basic medical services, coordinates, and, if required by the plan, authorizes referrals to specialists and hospitals." (Website of the USA Federal Government, 2004 — see References)

Primary Coverage

The term *primary coverage* is used to describe the insurance coverage/insurance company that receives the claim first when an individual is covered by more than one insurance plan.

Secondary Coverage

The term *secondary coverage* is used to describe the insurance coverage/insurance company that receives the claim after the first insurance company has processed the claim and made a payment. This occurs when an individual is covered by more than one insurance plan.

Subscriber

In managed care, a *subscriber* is defined as "an individual, agency, or employer that has contracted for services under a health plan". (*Mosby's Medical Dictionary*, 2002)

Usual, Customary, and Reasonable (UCR) Charges

"Conventional indemnity plans operate based on *usual, customary, and reasonable (UCR) charges*. UCR charges mean that the charge is the provider's usual fee for a service that does not exceed the customary fee in that geographic area, and is reasonable based on the circumstances. Instead of UCR charges, PPO plans often operate based on a negotiated (fixed) schedule of fees that recognize charges for covered services up to a negotiated fixed dollar amount." (Website of the USA Federal Government, 2004 — see References)

Waiting Period/Elimination Period

Waiting period or *elimination period* refers to a specific amount of time a new employee must wait before the employee and his or her family members are eligible for insurance benefits. Different companies have different rules regarding this issue; some companies have one-month waiting periods, while other companies can have three-month waiting periods. It is important to know up front what your company's policy is so you and your family are not without medical or dental benefits. If you need insurance coverage during the waiting period you can choose to elect COBRA benefits if you are eligible for them (see COBRA definition).

Helpful Tips

Listed below are tips that will help take some of the confusion and frustration out of dealing with payment and insurance issues.

Tip #1

When you choose which medical and dental insurance plan to go with, be sure you understand what the benefits and drawbacks to each plan are before you sign up (assuming you have a choice to sign up to begin with). If you don't understand enough about the plan you sign up for, you may end up paying more money out of pocket than you expected or you may not be able to see doctors you want to see and still use your plan. Knowing how an insurance plan works and what limitations there are before you sign up can help save you from these frustrations.

Your employer or group (if you go with group insurance) should be able to provide you with some comparison information regarding the different plans that are offered. This information should include information about: premiums due, copays, individual and family deductibles, individual and family out-of-pocket limits, individual lifetime maximums, coinsurance payments, etc.

It is also important to know if you can seek medical care from anyone or if you have to go to specific offices. Some plans let you go to any office, but you may pay more if that health care provider doesn't participate with your insurance plan (out-of-network). If you don't receive the answers to your questions from your employer or group, you can always contact directly the insurance company you are planning to go with and ask what the benefits are for your company. You will probably need to give the insurance company a specific group number that you can get from your employer, since insurance companies use these numbers when looking up benefits.

Generally, insurance plans that tend to have lower annual premiums, lower deductibles and lower out-of-pocket payments may also have less freedom of choice when it comes to where and who you can see as your health care providers.

Plans that cost you more generally allow you more freedom to see health care providers of your choice. Most people try to find a balance between cost and the freedom to seek their own that they can be happy with. Having said this, if you or a family member become seriously ill, having the freedom to find the best doctor to help you or your family member is much more important than saving some money with a less expensive health care plan. Costs for health care can be financed if necessary.

Tip #2

Always check that the office or hospital you are seeking care from participates with your insurance. You should ask this question before you schedule an appointment. Depending on your insurance plan and the office's response, you may not be eligible to be seen at the office expecting to use your insurance coverage. Some insurance plans require you to go only to certain offices. Asking if your insurance is accepted ahead of time will save you from wasting your time if you cannot be seen. Knowing whether you are receiving care from an in-network provider or an out-of-network provider can also make a big difference in what you may be responsible for financially. Insurance plans that distinguish between in-network and out-of-network providers encourage members to seek care in-network by having higher fees associated with out-of-network care. There is nothing wrong with seeking care out-of-network if you feel that is the best place for you to receive care, but you need to understand going out-of-network will end up costing you more money.

Tip #3

Take all of your insurance information with you when you seek medical or dental care. Wherever you go, the office will want to see your insurance card or information. Also it is a really good idea to know what your insurance benefits are before you go to an office. Knowing what you owe for routine office visits (primary care physician vs. specialist; in-network vs. out-of-network) and what percentage you may owe on procedures can be very helpful. Believe it or not there are some receptionists who will ask *you* what you owe for an office visit (especially the first time you visit the office). If you know your benefits, you can sometimes avoid overpaying or underpaying for your visit to the doctor.

Tip #4

If your insurance plan requires you to pay deductibles, coinsurance or copays, be sure to match your EOBs (Explanation of Benefits) from your insurance company with the paperwork you receive from your office visits, appointments, or hospital stays. While this is an extra step, it can help prevent you from paying too much. Information such as date of service, individual and total charges for services, amount you paid vs. amount your insurance expects you to pay, etc. should all be double-checked to ensure that the provider of services (i.e., doctor's office, laboratory, or hospital) information matches your insurance information. Mistakes at the provider's office or the insurance company are possible! These mistakes can cost you money if you do not find them and make some phone calls to have them corrected. If you have billing questions, make sure you find out the answers before you pay your portion of the bills.

Matching EOBs to services rendered is even more important when costly procedures are performed or when many services are delivered at the same time as in the case of a hospital stay. Hospital bills often don't list all the detailed services. Since you really need the detailed services to be able to match services provided to your insurance information, it's a good idea to speak with someone in the hospital's billing department. They should be able to provide you with an item-by-item list of services and supplies you received. Don't be surprised if you have to ask for this. This service is generally not offered to you unless you ask for it. If you have questions after receiving this information, don't pay your bills until you understand what you are paying for. Most billing departments are happy to answer your questions. Occasionally, someone even finds a procedure or prescription they are being billed for that they never even received.

Tip #5

If possible, get to know who is in charge of insurance/billing at the medical/dental offices where you seek care. While this is an extra step, it can help you when you need to have questions answered. Today there are many types of insurance plans and oftentimes the receptionist is not the person who handles the insurance paperwork. Knowing the right person to ask can save you time and frustration.

Tip #6

Ask for a pre-authorization or pre-certification before you have expensive medical or health care procedures done. Some offices and hospitals will do these routinely on costly services like surgery, but it's still important to make sure your insurance is aware of the procedure to be performed and that it is a covered service. Pre-authorizing or pre-certifying services can help you understand what fees you will be responsible for ahead of time. This way there will be no big surprises. No one wants to have an expensive procedure done only to find out that the insurance will not pay anything towards it. It doesn't hurt to confirm that this paperwork (pre-authorization or pre-certification) has been done with both your insurance company and the office or hospital where the procedure/service will be done prior to your appointment date.

Tip #7

Have patience about incoming bills and statements from your insurance company. If you have a number of procedures done, or many services done at the same time as in the case of surgery, you may see statements and bills coming in from many different sources over a long period of time. It's not unheard of to receive bills even six months to a year after the day the service was performed. It takes some organization, a bit of detective work, and a lot of patience sometimes to figure it all out.

Besides arriving at different times, multiple bills can come from many different sources for the same date of service. For example, if you were to visit an emergency room, you would receive bills from the hospital, of course, but you also may receive bills for the doctors you saw that might use an outside billing company. That means you might receive a bill from a company with a name you do not recognize with a service date as the same date you visited the emergency room. Sometimes it takes a phone call or two to figure out that the bill you have received is for the emergency room doctor who treated you.

In the case of a surgery, you may receive other bills. You could have separate bills from: the hospital, the anesthesiologist, the surgeon, physical therapy, etc. You need to stay organized, have a notebook or *My Medical Organizer* (see Chapter 5 — Organizing Your Care) available to organize the paperwork by service dates, and know which bills you have paid and which bills still have to be paid. Finally, you need to take a couple of deep breaths and try to relax when another bill arrives months later. Eventually the incoming bills will end.

Tip #8

If you are having difficulty making your health care payments, you need to ask the office or hospital if payment or installment plans are available. Oftentimes an office or hospital will be willing to work out a payment plan with you. After all, they would rather see regular payments being made than no payment at all. Most of the time you will not be offered these services up front, you will have to ask for them. Sometimes payment plans are available without interest, especially at larger facilities like hospitals. Other payment plans may require that a small amount of interest or installment fees be paid in addition to the balance owed. Usually there is a minimum payment due each month. It does pay to ask. You will never know what an office or hospital is willing to do to assist you in paying off your balance unless you ask!

Tip #9

It is also important to know what types of personal payment (i.e., cash, check, credit card) are accepted at the office, laboratory, or hospital you visit. Don't assume that everyone accepts credit cards, because every office doesn't — or they may not accept your specific card. It can be an embarrassing situation if you intend to pay by credit card at an office that only accepts cash or checks. Every time you make a payment by credit card a percentage of your payment must be paid to the credit card company by the office or facility accepting your payment. So, each time you pay by credit card the office or facility doesn't get to keep all of the payment you made. For this reason, many offices choose not to accept credit card payments. Play it safe and find out before a payment is due what type of payments the office, laboratory, or hospital will accept.

You should also keep in mind that unless you pay off your credit card balances each month, paying large medical bills by credit cards can be expensive. You could end up with a lot of extra interest on the balance carried from month to month. If you do not pay off your credit card balances each month it would be much smarter to set up a payment plan with the office or facility on a cash or check basis. As long as the office or facility is willing to work with you on a payment plan, you would probably be paying a lot less interest this way.

Tip #10

It is very important to keep track of and organize your medical and dental expenses. Medical/dental expenses that exceed 7.5 percent of your adjusted gross income can be used as an itemized deduction when figuring your taxes. You will not know if this deduction applies to you unless you keep track of your total medical/dental expenses for each tax year.

As an example, if your adjusted gross income is $20,000, you would be able to deduct paid medical/dental expenses that were over $1500 ($20,000 X .075). If you paid $4000 in medical/dental expenses for this particular tax year, you could claim $2500 ($4000 -$1500) in itemized deductions. If instead you only paid $800 in medical/dental expenses for the same tax year, you would not be able to deduct any of the expenses since they were less than the $1500 (7.5 percent of $20,000 adjusted gross income).

You can find out more information about deducting medical/dental expenses from your accountant or from Publication 502 from the Internal Revenue Service (Department of the Treasury, United States Government). Publication 502 can be found at the IRS website www.irs.gov/publications/p502/ar02.html

This website explains that keeping track of your medical/dental expenses means keeping a record of:

❖ The name and address of each person you paid, and

❖ The amount and date of each payment.

You should also keep a statement or itemized invoice showing the following information:

❖ What medical care was received.

❖ Who received the care.

❖ The nature and purpose of any other medical expenses.

❖ Who the other medical expenses were for.

❖ The amount of the other medical expenses and the date of payment.

This information is not sent with your tax return, but needs to be kept by you. Your accountant may need copies of the information as well.

In addition to knowing how to record the information about your deductions, you also need to know which medical/dental expenses can be deducted and which medical/dental expenses cannot be deducted. The IRS website listed previously can provide detailed information about deductible and non-deductible expenses. This detailed information is necessary when trying to decide if specific expenses are deductible or not. For example, certain expenses for weight loss programs like membership in a weight reduction group are deductible if they are considered treatment for a specific disease diagnosed by a physician (i.e., obesity, hypertension, or heart disease). Other weight loss expenses like membership dues at a gym are not deductible. If you are unsure if an expense is deductible, consult the IRS website or your accountant.

Examples of deductible medical/dental expenses listed at this website include:

Abortion	Braille books and magazines
Acupuncture	Capital expenses
Alcoholism	Car
Ambulance	Chiropractor
Artificial limb	Christian Science practitioner
Artificial teeth	Contact lenses
Autoette	Crutches
Bandages	Dental treatment
Breast reconstruction surgery	Diagnostic devices
Birth control pills	Disabled dependent care

Drug addiction

Drugs

Eyeglasses

Eye surgery

Fertility enhancement

Founder's fee

Guide dog or other animal

Health Institute

Health Maintenance
Organization (HMO)

Hearing aids

Home care

Home improvements

Hospital services

Insurance premiums

Laboratory fees

Lead-based paint removal

Learning disability

Legal fees

Lifetime care-advance
payments

Lodging

Long-term care

Meals

Medical conferences

Medical information plan

Medical services

Medicine

Mentally retarded (special home)

Nursing home

Nursing services

Operations

Optometrist

Organ donors

Osteopath

Oxygen

Prosthesis

Psychiatric care

Psychoanalysis

Psychologist

Special education

Sterilization

Stop-smoking programs

Surgery

Telephone

Television

Therapy

Transplants

Transportation

Trips

Tuition

Vasectomy

Vision correction surgery

Weight-loss program (depends
on type of expense — see IRS website)

Wheelchair

Wig

X-ray

Examples of non-deductible medical/dental expenses listed at this website include:

Baby sitting, child care, and nursing services for a normal, healthy baby	Household help
	Illegal operations and treatments
Controlled substances	Insurance premiums
Cosmetic surgery	Maternity clothes
Dancing lessons	Medical savings account (MSA)
Diaper service	Nonprescription drugs and medicines
Electrolysis or hair removal	Nutritional supplements
Funeral expenses	Personal use items
Future medical care	Swimming lessons
Hair transplant	Teeth whitening
Health club dues	Veterinary fees
Health coverage tax credit	Weight-loss program (depends on type of expense — see IRS website)

You need to develop your own method of keeping track of medical/dental expenses. Some people simply keep written notes, while others use their computers. Computer programs today that use a spreadsheet can make medical/dental expense record keeping much easier. Regardless of the system you choose to use, keep track of those expenses. You cannot take advantage of deducting the medical/dental expenses if you don't know what they total for any given tax year. Remember, tracking and recording medical/dental expenses that exceed 7.5 percent of your adjusted gross income can save you money in taxes through itemized deductions.

Reviewing Insurance Information

A completed example of the *Insurance Information* form for reviewing insurance information can be found on the next two pages. If your insurance company, group, or employer has already provided you with a chart of this information, you don't need to copy it all over again. If this is the case, the form on the next page is simply meant for you to make sure you understand these benefit topics. However, if you do not have all this information in one place, you can fill in this form. Either way, it is here to help you better understand your medical insurance policy or a specific claim. If you are unsure of areas of the form, you should contact your insurance company to have your questions answered. (For photocopying purposes, a blank *Insurance Information* form can be found in Appendix 1.)

Insurance Information *(page 1)*

Your Name: _IMA Smart Patient_

Today's Date: _May 1, 2004_

1. Name of your insurance company _Aetna PPO_

2. Are you covered by another insurance company?

(No)   If yes, the name is _____

Which company is primary? _____

secondary_____

(If you have more than one use a second page for the second company)

3. Identification information for your insurance:

Group# _987654_

I.D.# _123456789_

4. Information you need to know about your insurance:

Is there a **waiting period** before you can use your insurance?

No   (Yes)   If yes, how long? _1 month, but already past_
this amount of time

Premium amount (per month or per year) is _$90/mo. (for family)_

In-network **deductible** (individual/family) _$250/$500_

Out-of-network **deductible** (individual/family) _$750/$1500_

In-network **out-of-pocket limit** (individual/family) _$2000/$4000_

Out-of-network **out-of-pocket limit** (individual/family) _$3000/$6000_

In-network **lifetime maximum benefit** (individual) _$2 million_

Out-of-network **lifetime maximum benefit** (individual) _$2 million_

Insurance Information *(page 2)*

Copays/coinsurance (In-network/Out-of-network):

Office visit <u>$20 or ($40 specialist) in-network/</u>
<u>65% out-of-network</u>

Preventative testing <u>100% in-network/not covered out-of-network</u>

Well-child care <u>$25 in-network/not covered out-of-network</u>

Hospital stays <u>85% in-network/65% out-of-network</u>

Emergency room <u>$100 copay then covered at 100% in-network</u>
<u>$100 copy then covered at 100% out-of-network</u>

Other covered services <u>85% in-network/65% out-of-network</u>

Prescriptions: (No difference in-network or out-of-network)

1st tier <u>$10 copay</u>

2nd tier <u>$25 copay</u>

3rd tier <u>$40 copay</u>

Mail order Prescriptions:

1st tier <u>$10 copay</u>

2nd tier <u>$20 copay</u>

3rd tier <u>$35 copay</u>

Other notes: <u>Plan runs from January 1st to December 31st.</u>
<u>Must see PPO providers (in-network) or risk extra fees</u>

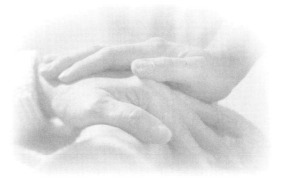

CHAPTER 7

Other Matters of Importance

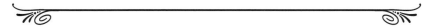

Unlike many of the areas in this book that can be taught by example, the following topics are more individual and require additional thought and planning on your part. This chapter will start you thinking about how the following matters may affect you:

- ✤ Finding time to do the looking out.

- ✤ Traveling for treatment.

- ✤ Other costs associated with medical care.

- ✤ Where to find support and comfort during the process.

- ✤ Decisions, decisions, decisions regarding your treatment.

- ✤ Proceeding with gusto can help your body fight illness.

- ✤ A review of the care steps.

- ✤ Finding peace of mind.

Finding Time

When you begin taking an active role in your own health care or that of a loved one, you may need to adjust your lifestyle and schedule to find the time to do it. Making the time, adjusting your daily activities, and working with a patient advocate, if you need one, may seem challenging at first. You may find it easier if you adopt some of the following suggestions, if applicable:

✤ Cut back on social activities.

✤ Find a sitter for your children.

✤ Cut back on your household work. If needed, hire a cleaning lady.

✤ If you work at home, do what has to be done, not everything that could be done.

✤ If you work outside the home, speak with your employer and let your boss know you have a personal/medical problem you need to work through. Most employers appreciate the heads up and are willing to help you if they can.

✤ Use personal time or vacation time you have accumulated at work.

✤ Let family and friends and/or your patient advocate help you free up more time.

When you sit down and think about it, you may find other creative ways to find time to research your disease or condition and get the treatment you so well deserve without unnecessary stress.

Traveling for Treatment

As you consider where to seek treatment, you will want to assess how far you are willing to travel for treatment. Having to travel long distances for appointments or treatment is more time consuming and requires more lifestyle adjustments. So think about the following questions before you decide:

❖ Would traveling create further hardships in your life?

❖ Do you need someone to watch your children, your spouse, or a parent?

❖ How would you get to your appointments (car, bus, plane, train)?

❖ Do you need someone to go with you to appointments?

❖ Do you have someone (family member or friend) who would be willing to travel with you?

❖ If the care center you are considering is far away, where will you stay (motel, hotel, with family or friends)? Some large hospitals and care centers do offer places for patients and family members to stay also.

❖ How often would you need to make the trip?

❖ Would you need to make the trip for a period of days, weeks, months, or years?

❖ Can you take enough time off from work (personal days, vacation, medical leave of absence)?

❖ What is the cost of traveling (parking, plane tickets, lodging, food, etc.)?

Most people would rather stay as close to home as possible for their treatment. This requires less time and usually offers more support from family and friends. However, if you have a rare disease or condition, or need very specialized care, then there may only be a few places in the country that can help you. In cases of serious medical conditions, you need to concentrate on finding the best place to be treated, not necessarily the most convenient. It's a good idea to work through the answers to the above questions with your patient advocate because they may have solutions you haven't thought of yet.

Other Costs

In a perfect world everyone would have access to the best medical care regardless of cost. The reality is that the cost of medical care increases every year. Some people have private insurance coverage, while others do not. Some have medical coverage through government programs such as Medicaid or Medicare. And others fall through the cracks and must rely on emergency care at city hospitals only.

Unfortunately, by the time you are diagnosed with a condition, it's probably too late to do anything about changing your medical coverage. The best you can do is to understand what your options are and use them to your best advantage. As discussed in Chapter 6, you need to understand your own situation. You may need to speak with your employee benefit representatives, insurance representatives, hospital billing staff, government agency representatives, etc. They will be able to help guide you through what benefits are available to you and what co-payments you will be responsible for.

However, there may be additional indirect costs (not covered by any medical plan) you need to consider as well:

❖ Less income if you have cut back your time at work or you are on medical leave or disability.

❖ Increased costs of child care.

❖ Increased costs of over-the-counter medications.

❖ Increased costs due to more co-pays and coinsurance.

❖ Costs associated with traveling to appointments (parking, plane tickets, lodging, etc.).

❖ Costs associated with researching your disease (Internet time, copies, phone calls, etc.).

Taking the time to think about these possible other costs can help prevent surprise bills later. Depending on how high your out-of-pocket costs are, you may have to find creative answers like finding a job you can do from home, having another family member increase their income, having another family member or friend loan you money, taking a loan from your retirement account, etc. Whatever options you consider, find out what the short-term and long-term risks are.

Support and Comfort

Anyone diagnosed with a serious medical disease or condition is going to need support and comfort. Support and comfort can come from many sources and the important thing is to find the combination that works for you. People often think of family and friends as the biggest sources of support and comfort. While this is probably true for most people, there are other sources as well.

Keep in mind that people are always willing to help out in the beginning, but as time goes on it becomes harder for people to continue the same level of support. If you're lucky enough to find people who are willing and able to go the distance with you, then you are truly blessed. Sources of support and comfort you may want to consider are:

✤ Family.

✤ Friends.

✤ Church.

✤ Support group (phone buddy, local meeting, Internet buddy, etc.).

✤ Hobby (whatever you can still do that makes you happy).

✤ Relaxation (music, meditation, yoga etc.).

✤ Professional help (psychologists, psychiatrists, social workers, etc.).

Ultimately, each person finds his or her own support network and ways to find comfort.

Decisions, Decisions, Decisions!

After your diagnosis has been confirmed and you've researched your disease or condition and sought additional opinions; it's time to make some decisions. As long as you are of sound mind, the important decisions about your care are yours to determine. Although your patient advocate, family, friends, and other professionals can all make their opinions known to you, you have the final decisions to make about your care and quality of life. You get to decide what treatments you will undergo, what treatments you don't want, and how you choose to live the rest of your life.

Once you've made your decisions, be prepared for mixed reactions from family and friends. If you are lucky, most of them will be supportive and willing to help with whatever is necessary. However, some of your family and friends may not agree with your decisions. The most you can hope for is that the family and friends who aren't in agreement with you won't hinder you from proceeding forward in whatever way you choose.

Let your loved ones know that your decisions are based on what you feel is best for you in the long run. Accept help and support wherever it's offered and recognize the fact that you can't please everyone. Regarding your medical condition, look out for yourself first.

Proceeding with Gusto

Once you've found the best workable solution, it's time to move forward. Whatever you decide to do, there comes a time when you must "go for it". This means that you don't go with your decisions halfheartedly, but rather with 100 percent effort, energy, and belief. If you decide to fight a deadly disease, then fight with all you've got — give 100 percent. If you decide not to fight a deadly disease and you want to live the rest of your life as fully as possible, then give this effort your best. If you move forward with anything less than this, you are just cheating yourself. Now is the time to be your own best friend. It's important to believe in your decisions and make a commitment to see them through.

One of the reasons it's so important to believe in your decisions fully is that there is a strong mind-body connection. The mind-body connection refers to the fact that your brain (and nervous system) communicates with the rest of your body. While there is still a great deal unknown about how this connection works, it's clear that the state of one's mind can have a large impact on one's bodily health and vice-versa. Researchers have found that the brain is actually able to produce substances that can improve your health ("The Mind-Body

Connection" from www.webmd.com). The brain can create:

- ❖ Endorphins (natural painkillers).

- ❖ Gamma globulin (fortify your immune system).

- ❖ Interferon (fight infections, viruses, and even cancer).

- ❖ Combinations of these and other substances
  (for tailor-made prescriptions for whatever ails you).

The substance your brain produces depends in part upon your thoughts, feelings, and expectations. Negative attitudes and expectations (about an illness or life in general) may result in your brain not producing enough of the substance your body needs to heal. The opposite is also true, with positive attitudes and expectations more likely to have your brain produce sufficient amounts of the substance that will boost your body's healing power ("The Mind-Body Connection" from www.webmd.com).

While it's true that the mind affects the body — through the production of chemicals — it is also true that the body can affect the mind. A bodily injury or illness can cause long-term physical stress that can lead to chemical imbalances in the brain. These chemical imbalances may lead to depression and/or other mental health problems ("The Mind-Body Connection" from www.webmd.com).

Other studies are investigating the effects of stress on the immune system. While more study is needed, there is evidence that moody, nervous, and tense people may have weaker immune responses than their calmer, cooler counterparts ("Neurotic People May Have Weaker Immune Systems" from www.webmd.com). Although researchers are not sure how stress affects the immune system, people who are more psychologically or physically stressed often have elevated levels of the stress hormone cortisol. Cortisol is a known immune system suppressant.

While much more work needs to be done in the area of mind-body connection research, it's clear that there is an important and powerful connection. Doing all you can to positively influence this connection is in your best interest. Mind-body relaxation techniques have been developed to positively affect this connection. Examples of mind-body relaxation techniques include deep breathing, progressive muscle relaxation, guided imagery or visualization, meditation, yoga, tai chi, and even listening to music or enjoying nature. Health care providers that recommend these practices believe that "using mind-body techniques can enhance your quality of life, lessen pain, and may extend your longevity." These types of practices are being recommended for patients with serious illnesses like cancer ("Mind-Body Medicine for Cancer" from www.webmd.com).

Even without scientific studies, many people recognize that those who believe they feel better or they'll get better often do get better; while people who believe only the worst will happen often become worse. It is your life to do the best you can with it. It is up to you to make the most out of the time you have — both physically and mentally.

Care Steps

This section is designed to show you how different steps presented in this book can be sequenced together. Completing these steps will assist you in better organizing your care and help you keep track of where you are on your medical journey.

Some of the steps should be done routinely before you encounter a serious diagnosis. The more organized you are to begin with, the easier and faster it will be to get a plan for after the diagnosis. These routine steps are called "General Care Steps" and are listed below. All of these steps were discussed earlier in this book. Page numbers have been listed after each step in case you want to review what was presented. While many of these steps are ongoing, the checklist boxes can be used initially to make sure you are doing each step. These steps are general guidelines; you may need to adjust them to fit your particular situation. Once you have a system in place, it's important to update it as soon as you have new information. These steps will not be of value unless they are updated with your current medical information.

General Care Steps

1. ❑ Patient Advocate (form)   pg. 239

2. ❑ Medical Alert Information   pg. 21

3. ❑ My Medications (form)   pg. 255

4. ❑ My New Rx Medication (form)   pg. 256

5. ❑ Health History (form)   pg. 258

6. ❑ Organize Your Care   pg. 164
   (notebook or *My Medical Organizer*)

7. ❑ Collect Medical Information   pg. 32

8. ❑ Insurance Information (form)   pg. 264

Other steps can be taken after you have been given a diagnosis. These steps are listed on the next page and should be performed after the General Care Steps have been completed. If you have not had the time to finish the General Care Steps, you may have to work on each step as you are able to. Similarly, you may review information about a particular step by returning to the appropriate page number. You will notice that some of the After the Diagnosis Care Steps also appear under General Care Steps. This is because there may be new information as a result of a new diagnosis. An example of this would be a new medication added or new insurance information related to a specific diagnosis. Again, this list is meant to be a checklist guideline for your use. You may need to adapt it for your particular situation.

After the Diagnosis Care Steps

For photocopying purposes, these checklists and all the forms found in this book can be found in Appendix 1. Take advantage of them and use them to get organized.

Finding Peace of Mind

Peace of mind comes from being comfortable with your decisions. In order to find peace of mind you need to make your decisions based on all the information available to you.

Remember, smart patients will use their skills along with the information they have gathered to help them make the best decisions. So, once you have (S) sought help, (M) made decisions, plans and become organized, (A) asked questions, (R) completed research and investigation, it is time to (T) trust your instincts. Trusting your instincts means listening to that little voice inside you that lets you know you have done or will do the right thing. Be a SMART patient and use the information in this book to help you look out for yourself or a loved one. This will enable you to make the best decisions along with your health care providers.

At the end of the day, trusting your instincts and knowing you have done all you could do along your medical journey should help you find your peace of mind. Best wishes to you on your medical journey. Good Luck!

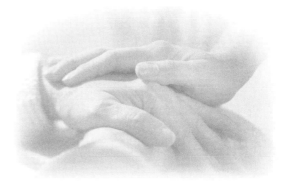

Appendix 1

Forms

This section contains all of the forms found in this book. Please do not write directly on these forms (especially if this is not your book)! If you write on these pages, you will lose the ability to use the forms again and again through photocopying.

These blank forms are placed all together so you can easily photocopy them and fill in the answers appropriate for you. You will inevitably find yourself using some forms more than others. You might want to consider making extra photocopies of the forms you use most often. This can save you a trip back to your photocopying site unless you have the ability to make copies at home.

These forms are meant to help you, so please use them!

Patient Advocate(s)
for

_____
(Your Name)

Effective as of _____
(Date)

First Advocate (Primary)

Name: _____

Address: _____

Address: _____

Phone #: _____

Phone #: _____

Second Advocate (Secondary)

Name: _____

Address: _____

Address: _____

Phone #: _____

Phone #: _____

Location of legal papers: _____

_____

_____

_____

_____

Questions to Ask after the Diagnosis
Part I — Initial Questions *(page 1)*

Your Name: _____

Doctor's Name: _____

Doctor's Phone #: _____

Today's Date: _____

1. What are your main symptoms (problems)? _____

_____

_____

_____

_____

_____

2. Circle all words that describe your disease or illness.

Mild   Moderate   Severe

Acute   Chronic

Benign   Malignant

Stage I   Stage II   Stage III   Stage IV

3. What is the name of your *suspected* disease or condition? _____

_____

_____

_____

_____

_____

Questions to Ask after the Diagnosis
Part I — Initial Questions *(page 2)*

4. Second/third opinion recommended?

Specialist? _____

Type/whom/when? _____

Therapist (physical/ psychological/occupational, etc.)?_____

_____

Type/whom/when? _____

5. How much time do I have to make treatment decisions?

_____Days _____Weeks _____Months

6. Initial treatment recommendations:

Additional testing needed (ex: blood tests, x-rays, CAT scan, MRI, biopsy, etc.)?

What test? _____

When? _____

What test? _____

When? _____

What test? _____

When? _____

Additional office visits?

Doctor:_____

When? _____

Doctor:_____

When? _____

Doctor:_____

When? _____

Questions to Ask after the Diagnosis
Part I — Initial Questions *(page 3)*

Possible treatment options:

Medication only? _____

Surgery? _____

_____

Radiation? _____

Chemotherapy? _____

Therapy (physical/ psychological/occupational, etc.)? _____

_____

Other? _____

Medications needed?

What? _____

How much, when? _____

_____

What? _____

How much, when? _____

_____

Changes needed?

Diet? _____

_____

Exercise? _____

Habit cessation (smoking/alcohol/drugs, etc.)? _____

Other? _____

Questions to Ask after the Diagnosis
Part I — Initial Questions *(page 4)*

Note: Initial treatment recommendations should be followed with specific treatment recommendations as soon as enough information is available — see form, *Questions to Ask after the Diagnosis, Part II — Specific Treatment Recommendations.*

Referral needed?

Specialist? _____

_____

Type/whom/when? _____

_____

Therapist (physical/psychological/occupational, etc.)? _____

_____

Type/whom/when _____

_____

7. Collecting medical information

Do you have copies of?

_____Diagnosis   _____Test results   _____Letters

_____Treatment recommendations   _____Other

8. Other questions: _____

_____

_____

_____

_____

_____

Questions to Ask after the Diagnosis

Part II — Specific Treatment Recommendations *(page 1)*

Your Name: _____

Doctor's Name: _____

Doctor's Specialty: _____

Doctor's Phone #: _____

Today's Date: _____

1. What are your main symptoms (problems)? _____

_____

_____

_____

_____

_____

2. Circle all words that describe your disease or illness.

    Mild   Moderate   Severe

    Acute   Chronic

    Benign   Malignant

    Stage I   Stage II   Stage III   Stage IV

3. What is the name of your *suspected* disease or condition? _____

_____

_____

_____

_____

_____

Questions to Ask after the Diagnosis

Part II — Specific Treatment Recommendations *(page 2)*

4. Additional testing needed (ex: blood tests, x-rays, CAT scan, MRI, biopsy, etc.)?

   What test? _____

   When? _____

   What test? _____

   When? _____

   What test? _____

   When? _____

5. **Additional office visits?**

   Doctor:_____

   When? _____

   Doctor:_____

   When? _____

6. **Results of additional testing?**

   What test? _____

   Result? _____

   _____

   What test? _____

   Result? _____

   _____

   What test? _____

   Result? _____

   _____

7. **What is the *exact* name of your disease or condition after additional testing?**

   _____

   _____

   _____

Questions to Ask after the Diagnosis
Part II — Specific Treatment Recommendations *(page 3)*

8. How much time do I have to make treatment decisions?

_____Days   _____Weeks   _____Months

9. Specifics about your treatment option(s):

<u>OPTION #1:</u>

Recommended treatment: _____

_____

_____

Length of treatment: _____

_____

_____

Medications needed?

What?_____

How much, when? _____

_____

_____

What?_____

How much, when? _____

_____

_____

What?_____

How much, when? _____

_____

_____

Questions to Ask after the Diagnosis

Part II — Specific Treatment Recommendations *(page 4)*

Additional testing/monitoring needed? _____

_____

_____

Side effects of treatment: _____

_____

Risks of treatment: _____

_____

_____

_____

Short-term prognosis: _____

_____

Long-term prognosis: _____

_____

_____

Is treatment covered by my insurance?

   No

   Yes – If yes, at what percentage(s)? _____

   _____

   Other payment questions (see *Insurance Form* in Chapter 6): _____

   _____

   _____

   _____

Questions to Ask after the Diagnosis

Part II — Specific Treatment Recommendations *(page 5)*

<u>OPTION #2:</u>

Recommended treatment: _____

_____

_____

Length of treatment: _____

_____

_____

Medications needed?

  What? _____

  How much, when? _____

_____

_____

  What? _____

  How much, when? _____

_____

_____

  What? _____

  How much, when? _____

_____

_____

Additional testing/monitoring needed? _____

_____

_____

Questions to Ask after the Diagnosis
Part II — Specific Treatment Recommendations *(page 6)*

Side effects of treatment: _____

_____

Risks of treatment: _____

_____

_____

_____

Short-term prognosis: _____

_____

Long-term prognosis: _____

_____

_____

Is treatment covered by my insurance?

    No

    Yes – If yes, at what percentage(s)? _____

    _____

    Other payment questions (see *Insurance Form* in Chapter 6): _____

    _____

    _____

    _____

    _____

Questions to Ask after the Diagnosis

Part II — Specific Treatment Recommendations *(page 7)*

OPTION #3:

Recommended treatment: _____

_____

_____

Length of treatment: _____

_____

_____

Medications needed?

What?_____

How much, when? _____

_____

_____

What?_____

How much, when? _____

_____

_____

What?_____

How much, when? _____

_____

_____

Additional testing/monitoring needed? _____

_____

_____

Questions to Ask after the Diagnosis

Part II — Specific Treatment Recommendations *(page 8)*

Side effects of treatment: _____

_____

Risks of treatment: _____

_____

_____

_____

Short-term prognosis: _____

_____

Long-term prognosis: _____

_____

_____

Is treatment covered by my insurance?

No

Yes – If yes, at what percentage(s)? _____

_____

Other payment questions (see *Insurance Form* in Chapter 6): _____

_____

_____

_____

_____

Questions to Ask after the Diagnosis

Part II — Specific Treatment Recommendations *(page 9)*

10. What treatment option do *you* think is in my best interest? _____

_____

_____

_____

_____

_____

11. Without any treatment, what is most likely to happen? _____

_____

_____

_____

How long will it take for these things to happen? _____

12. Treatment option _____ (fill in number) **was recommended to me by another doctor.**

Why do you think treatment option _____ (fill in number) is better?

_____

13. Do you offer/recommend a treatment that is unavailable elsewhere?

_____

_____

_____

14. Is there another treatment only available elsewhere for my condition?

_____

Questions to Ask after the Diagnosis
Part II — Specific Treatment Recommendations *(page 10)*

15. If I start treatment with you, will you follow my care or will other doctors help? How so? _____

_____

_____

_____

_____

_____

16. Who coordinates my care with other doctors and medical providers?

_____

_____

17. Who do I call and how do I reach them if I have a problem during treatment?

_____

_____

_____

_____

What number do I call if I have a problem outside of regular office hours?

_____

_____

18. How soon should treatment begin? _____

_____

_____

Questions to Ask after the Diagnosis

Part II — Specific Treatment Recommendations *(page 11)*

19. Can treatment be started quickly? _____

_____

20. What do I need to do to get started? _____

_____

_____

_____

_____

21. Collecting medical information

    I would like copies of:

    _____Diagnosis   _____Test results   _____Letters

    _____Treatment recommendations   _____Other

22. Other questions: _____

_____

_____

_____

_____

_____

_____

_____

_____

_____

My Medications

Your Name: _____

Doctor's Name / Phone #: _____

Pharmacy's Name / Phone #: _____

Today's Date: _____

1. Current medication(s) (name, strength, form, how often taken, when started):

Name	Strength	Form	How often	When started

2. Allergy(allergies) and reaction(s)(what happened, when): _____

_____

_____

_____

_____

3. Bad non-allergic reaction(s) to a medication(s) (medication & what happened):

_____

_____

My New Rx Medication *(page 1)*

Your Name: _____

Doctor's Name: _____

Doctor's Phone #: _____

Today's Date: _____

1. Name, strength and form of new medication (be specific):_____

_____

_____

2. Amount of medication given per prescription (oz., # of pills, etc.):_____

_____

_____

3. Instructions for taking the medication:

Take by mouth   Apply to problem area

Do not chew   Avoid exposure to sunlight

Be careful about rising too fast after lying down

Take with food   Take on an empty stomach

_____

Avoid alcohol   Store: In the refrigerator   At room temperature

Avoid _____foods or _____ medicines within

_____hours of taking this medication.

Take in the morning   Take at bedtime

Once/day   Twice/day   Three times/day   Four times/day

My New Rx Medication *(page 2)*

4. Is a generic version of the medicine all right to use?

   No   Yes

5. How long will I need to be on this medicine?_____

_____

_____

_____

6. Are there refills available?

   No   Yes _____times

   Can I call your office if I need refills or will I need another appointment

   with you? _____

_____

_____

_____

_____

7. Do I need to have my blood checked while on this medicine?

   If yes, how often? _____

_____

_____

_____

_____

_____

_____

Health History *(page 1)*

Your Name: _____

Today's Date: _____

Please answer **yes** *or* **no** *to the following questions
and explain all answers:*

1. Are you in good health?_____

_____

_____

2. Are you currently seeing a physician? If yes, for what reason? _____

_____

_____

3. Have you ever been hospitalized? If yes, when and why? _____

_____

_____

_____

_____

4. Have you ever had surgery? If yes, when and what kind? _____

_____

_____

5. Have you ever had a blood transfusion? If yes, when and why? _____

_____

_____

Health History *(page 2)*

6. Have you had any change in your health in the past 5 years? _____

_____

_____

7. Are you allergic to any medication or substance? If yes, provide a specific name (if possible) and list what reaction you had._____

_____

_____

_____

8. Have you had any reaction to a local or general anesthesia? If yes, provide a specific name (if possible) and list what reaction you had.

_____

_____

9. Do you take any prescription or non-prescription drugs, medicines, or supplements (vitamins/herbs)? If yes, provide specific name, strength, form, how often taken, and when the drug/medicine/supplement was started.

_____

_____

_____

_____

10. Did you <u>recently</u> <u>stop</u> taking any prescription or non-prescription drugs, medicines, or pills? If yes, why did you stop?

_____

_____

Health History *(page 3)*

11. **Do you have any of the following diseases, illnesses or medical problems (please circle yes or no):**

yes	no	Abnormal bleeding	yes	no	Drug abuse
yes	no	AIDS/ARC	yes	no	Emotional problems
yes	no	Allergies	yes	no	Endocrine disturbance
yes	no	Anemia	yes	no	Epilepsy
yes	no	Ankle swelling	yes	no	Excessive thirst
yes	no	Arthritis	yes	no	Excessive weight loss
yes	no	Asthma	yes	no	Fainting spells
yes	no	Auto accident injury	yes	no	Frequent sore throats
yes	no	Behavorial problems	yes	no	Frequent urination
yes	no	Birth defects	yes	no	Growth disturbances
yes	no	Bone disease	yes	no	Hearing problems
yes	no	Brain illness	yes	no	Heart disease
yes	no	Breathing problems	yes	no	Heart murmur
yes	no	Bruise easily	yes	no	Hemodialysis
yes	no	Cancer	yes	no	Hemophilia
yes	no	Chemotherapy	yes	no	Hepatitis
yes	no	Chest pain	yes	no	Herpes (cold sore)
yes	no	Chronic pain	yes	no	High blood pressure
yes	no	Convulsions	yes	no	HIV
yes	no	Diabetes	yes	no	Injured during sports
yes	no	Dizziness	yes	no	Intravenous injections

(continued from previous page)

yes	no	Jaundice	yes	no	Rheumatic fever
yes	no	Kidney disease	yes	no	Rickets
yes	no	Liver disease	yes	no	Scarlet fever
yes	no	Low blood pressure	yes	no	Severe headaches
yes	no	Lung disease	yes	no	Shortness of breath
yes	no	Menstrual problems	yes	no	Skin rashes or sores
yes	no	Mental problems	yes	no	Stomach problems
yes	no	Nervous condition	yes	no	Stroke
yes	no	Pacemaker	yes	no	Swollen glands
yes	no	Persistent cough	yes	no	Thyroid disease
yes	no	Persistent diarrhea	yes	no	Tobacco use any form
yes	no	Persistent fever	yes	no	Tuberculosis
yes	no	Persistent tiredness	yes	no	Ulcers
yes	no	Pregnancy	yes	no	Venereal disease
yes	no	Prosthetic heart valve	yes	no	Vision problems
yes	no	Prosthetic joint	yes	no	Vitamin deficiency
yes	no	Radiation therapy			

12. Are their any medical problems that run in your family? If yes, what are they?

_____

_____

_____

_____

_____

What to Ask When Calling for the Other Opinion Appointments *(page 1)*

Your Name: _____

Doctor's Name: _____

Doctor's Phone #: _____

Who You Spoke With: _____

Today's Date: _____

1. **Is the doctor accepting new patients?**

   Yes   No

2. **Does the doctor accept your insurance?**

   Yes   No

3. **How long will I have to wait for the first appointment?**

   _____Days   _____Weeks   _____Months

   (Is your doctor comfortable with you waiting this long to be seen? Yes   No)

4. **What medical records does the office need? When are they needed?**

   ____Blood reports   ____Doctor's referral(s) and/or letter(s)

   ____X-rays reports   ____Actual x-ray films

   ____CAT scan reports   ____Actual CAT scan films

   ____MRI scan reports   ____Actual MRI scan films

   ____Ultrasound reports   ____Actual ultrasound films

   ____Biopsy reports   ____Pathology slides needed (from biopsy)

   ____Health history form (if sent to you by the new office/completed by you)

   ____Payment/Insurance form (if sent to you by the new office/completed by you)

What to Ask When Calling for
the Other Opinion Appointments *(page 2)*

____Other items needed _____

_____

_____

When are records needed?   ASAP (before appointment is made)?

                                   Or bring all items to first appointment?

5. Is any additional testing needed before you are seen?

No   If Yes, then what _____

_____

6. How long can I expect to be at the first appointment?

_____Minutes   _____Hours

7. Questions about location, directions or access to the building?

Will a map be sent?   Yes   No   If No, then how will I get there?

_____

_____

Is the office or facility handicap accessible?   Yes   No

8. Questions for your particular situation: _____

_____

_____

_____

_____

_____

Insurance Information *(page 1)*

Your Name: _____

Today's Date: _____

1. **Name of your insurance company** _____

2. **Are you covered by another insurance company?**

   No   If yes, the name is _____

   Which company is primary? _____

   secondary_____

   (If you have more than one use a second page for the second company)

3. **Identification information for your insurance:**

   Group# _____

   I.D.# _____

4. **Information you need to know about your insurance:**

   Is there a **waiting period** before you can use your insurance?

   No   Yes   If yes, how long?_____

   _____

   Premium amount (per month or per year) is _____

   In-network **deductible** (individual/family)_____

   Out-of-network **deductible** (individual/family) _____

   In-network **out-of-pocket limit** (individual/family) _____

   Out-of-network **out-of-pocket limit** (individual/family) _____

   In-network **lifetime maximum benefit** (individual) _____

   Out-of-network **lifetime maximum benefit** (individual) _____

Insurance Information *(page 2)*

Copays/coinsurance (In-network/Out-of-network):

Office visit _____

_____

Preventative testing _____

Well-child care _____

Hospital stays _____

Emergency room_____

_____

Other covered services_____

Prescriptions:

1st tier _____

2nd tier _____

3rd tier_____

Mail order Prescriptions:

1st tier_____

2nd tier _____

3rd tier_____

Other notes:_____

_____

_____

_____

_____

General Care Steps

After the Diagnosis Care Steps

1. ❏ The Diagnosis — pg. 27

2. ❏ Collect New Medical Information — pg. 32

3. ❏ Questions to Ask after the Diagnosis — pg. 240
   Part I — Initial Questions (form)

4. ❏ Questions to Ask after the Diagnosis — pg. 244
   Part II — Specific Treatment
   Recommendations (form)

5. ❏ Understand Basic Terms — pg. 58
   For Your Diagnosis

6. ❏ Understand Your Test Results — pg. 85

7. ❏ My New Rx Medication (form) — pg. 256

8. ❏ Research Your Diagnosis — pg. 143

9. ❏ Continue with Recommended Care — pg. 162

10. ❏ Add Updates to Organize Your Care — pg. 164
    (notebook or *My Medical Organizer*)

11. ❏ Seek Second/Third Opinions — pg. 175

12. ❏ What to Ask When Calling for — pg. 262
    Other Opinion Appointments (form)

13. ❏ Insurance Information (form) — pg. 264

14. ❏ Other Matters of Importance — pg. 225

15. ❏ Care Steps — pg. 233

16. ❏ Finding Peace of Mind — pg. 236

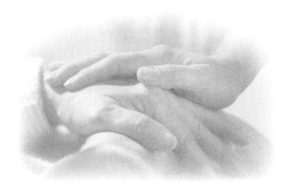

Appendix 2

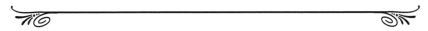

References

Books & Periodicals

America's Top Doctors. 2nd ed. New York: Castle Connolly, 2002; iii-viii.

Balas, EA. Information Systems Can Prevent Errors and Improve Quality. (Comment). *Journal of the American Medical Informatics Association* 2001; 8(4): 398-9.

Bates DW, Spell N, Cullen DJ, et al. The Costs of Adverse Drug Events in Hospitalized Patients. Adverse Drug Events Prevention Study Group. *JAMA* 1997; 277(4): 307-11.

Brodin, MB. *The Encyclopedia of Medical Tests*. New York: Simon & Schuster, Inc., 1997: 32-33, 68-69, 128-29, 157-58, 161-62, 266-67, 290-91, 314-15, 435-36, 474-75.

Centers for Disease Control and Prevention (National Center for Health Statistics). Births and Deaths; Preliminary Data for 1998. 1999. *National Vital Statistics Reports*. Washington, D.C.: Department of Health and Human Services.

Chassin MR. Assessing Strategies for Quality Improvement. *Health Aff* (Millwood) 1997; 16(3): 151-61.

Clark CM, Fradkin JE, Hiss RG, et. Al. Promoting Early Diagnosis and Treatment of Type 2 Diabetes: The National Diabetes Education Program. *JAMA* 2000; 284(3): 363-5.

Hobson, K. Doctors Vanish From View. *U.S. News & World Report* 2005; 138(4): 48-53.

Hooley JR, Whitacre, RJ. *A Self-Instructional Guide: Medications Used in Oral Surgery*. 3rd ed. Seattle: Stoma Press, Inc., 1984: 27.

Institute of Medicine. *To Err is Human: Building a Safer Health System*. Kohn LT, Corrigan JM, and Donaldson MS, eds. Washington D.C.: National Academy Press, 2000.

Institute of Medicine. *Care Without Coverage: Too Little, Too Late*. Washington, D.C.: National Academy Press, 2002.

Institute of Medicine. *Fostering Rapid Advances in Health Care: Learning from System Demonstrations*. Corrigan JM, Greiner A, and Erickson SM, eds. Washington D.C.; National Academy Press, 2003a.

Institute of Medicine. *Health Professions Education: A Bridge to Quality*. Greiner AC, and Knebel E, eds. Washington D.C.: National Academy Press, 2003b.

Institute of Medicine. *Priority Areas for National Action: Transforming Health Care Quality*. Adams K, and Corrigan JM, eds. Washington D.C.: National Academy Press, 2003c.

Legorreta AP, Liu X, Saher CA, and Jatulis DE. Variation in Managing Asthma: Experience at the Medical Group Level in California. *Am J Manag Care* 2000; 6(4): 445-53.

McBride P, Schrott HG, Plane MB, Underbakke G., and Brown RL. Primary Care Practice Adherence to National Cholesterol Education Program Guidelines for Patients with Coronary Heart Disease. *Arch Intern Med* 1998; 158(11): 1238-44.

McGlynn, EA, Asch SM, Adams J, et al. The Quality of Health Care Delivered to Adults in the United States. *N Engl J Med* 2003; 348: 2635-45.

Mosby's Medical Dictionary. 6th ed. St. Louis: Mosby, Inc., 2002: 8, 29, 66, 92, 94, 97, 103, 107-08, 112, 116, 122, 135, 147, 193, 206, 247, 252, 260, 266, 268-69, 271, 277, 292, 297, 307, 316, 351, 361, 372, 410, 418, 420, 424, 461, 466, 482-83, 495-6, 503, 511, 515, 532, 560-63, 580, 582, 585, 589, 591, 593, 597, 604, 639, 709, 724, 736, 771, 785, 793, 797, 841, 844, 849-50, 852-53, 858-60, 875, 890, 894, 905, 911, 917, 927, 930, 974, 978, 1010, 1018,1030, 1032, 1046, 1064, 1066, 1068, 1087, 1101, 1135, 1165, 1167, 1176, 1178, 1197, 1206-07, 1213, 1215, 1219, 1224, 1236, 1249, 1251, 1271, 1274, 1294, 1299, 1309, 1313, 1317-18, 1339, 1353, 1359, 1361, 1366-67, 1370-71,1375, 1388, 1400, 1409, 1417-18, 1420-21, 1427, 1434, 1438, 1457, 1460, 1481, 1487, 1499, 1506, 1621-22, 1624, 1643, 1648, 1655, 1659, 1661, 1673, 1692, 1704, 1718, 1724, 1740, 1763, 1774, 1781, 1783-84, 1798, 1856-59, 1861, 1864-67.

Ni H, Nauman DJ, and Hershberger RE. Managed Care and Outcomes of Hospitalization Among Elderly Patients with Congestive Heart Failure. *Arch Intern Med* 1998; 158(11): 1231-6.

Pagana KD, and Pagana, TJ. *Mosby's Manual of Diagnostic and Laboratory Tests.* 2nd ed. St. Louis: Mosby, Inc., 2002: 13-17.

Perez-Stable EJ, and Fuentes-Afflick E. Role of Clinicians in Cigarette Smoking Prevention. *West J Med* 1998; 169(1): 23-9.

Pope, E. Second-Class Care: Discrimination Against Older Patients Still Permeates Nation's Health Care System. *AARP Bulletin* Nov. 2003; Vol:44, No. 10: 6-8.

Querna, E, The Druggist is In. *U.S. News & World Report* 2005; 138(4):60.

Samas GP, Matchar DB, Goldstein LB, et al. Quality of Anticoagulation Management Among Patients with Atrial Fibrillation: Results of a Review of Medical Records from 2 Communities. *Arch Intern Med* 2000; 160(7): 967-73.

Smith, I. *Dr. Ian Smith's Guide to Medical Websites*. New York: Atrandom.com Books, 2001: xii, 3-6.

Stedman's Medical Dictionary. 24th ed. Baltimore: Williams & Wilkins, 1982: 717, 1145, 1677-78.

Steinberg, EP. Improving the Quality of Care — Can We Practice What We Preach? *N Engl J Med* 2003; 348: 2681-83.

Thomas EJ, Studdert DM, Burstin HR, et al. Incidence and Types of Adverse Events and Negligent Care in Utah and Colorado. (Comment). *Medical Care* 2000; 38(3): 261-71.

Thomas EJ, Studdert DM, Newhouse BIW, et al. Costs of Medical Injuries in Utah and Colorado. *Inquiry* 1999; 36(3):255-64.

Merriam-Webster's Collegiate Dictionary. 11th ed. Springfield: Merriam-Webster, Incorporated, 2004: 13, 798, 866, 1140, 1302, 1353.

Young AS, Klap R, Sherbourne CD, and Wells KB. The Quality of Care for Depressive and Anxiety Disorders in the United States. *Arch Gen Psychiatry* 2001; 58(1):55-61.

Websites

Alliance for Aging Research
"Ageism: How Health Care Fails the Elderly"
www.agingresearch.org/brochures/ageism/index.cfm

IRS (Department of Treasury, United States Government),
www.irs.gov/publications/p502/ar02.html

MedicAlert®,
www.medicalert.org

U.S. News & World Report,
www.usnews.com

USA Federal Government,
www.bls.gov/ncs/ebs/sp/healthterms.pdf

United States Pharmacopeia,
www.usp.org

WebMDHealth,
www.webmd.com

Continue Your Medical Journey with
My Medical Organizer

The Practical Companion to *After the Diagnosis*

My Medical Organizer is the next step to take after reading this book. The organizer is based on the ideas presented in Chapter 5 of *After the Diagnosis* and *it can save you both time and energy*. Using *My Medical Organizer* allows you to immediately start organizing your medical care instead of spending valuable time searching for and purchasing all the items from scratch.

My Medical Organizer contains:

✤ 3-Ring Binder for Easy Updating and Additions

✤ 16 Dividers with Printed Tabs

✤ Over 120 Pages of Text and Forms

✤ Yearly Insert Calendars — 2005 to 2010

✤ 12-Month Calendar Forms

✤ The *Right* Questions to Ask Medical Providers

✤ Appointment/Business Card Holders

✤ Pocket Holders

✤ Appendix Containing All the Forms for Ease of Photocopying

Get *My Medical Organizer* and start organizing *your* medical care today! It really is one of the best ways you can look out for yourself or a loved one!

My Medical Organizer may be purchased by visiting:
www.books2helpyou.com
or by calling toll-free **877-892-6657 (877-89BOOKS)**.

For More Information...

www.books2helpyou.com

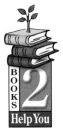

Published by:
Books 2 Help You, LLC
P.O. Box 130
Hartland, MI 48353
Phone: (877) 892-6657